FASTING FOR THE CURE OF DISEASE

BY
DR. LINDA BURFIELD HAZZARD

DIGITAL NINJAS MEDIA, INC.

Fasting For The Cure Of Diease: Published by Digital Ninjas Media, Inc. Printed in the United States of America. Originally published Physical Culture Publishing Co., New York City in 1908. This book is understood to reside in the public domain, as its legal copyright terms have expired, for open & free use in the United States of America. For further information, please address Digital Ninjas Media, Inc. [www.digitalninjasmedia.com].

Digital Ninjas Logos Copyright 2010-2016 Digital Ninjas Media, Inc. All Rights Reserved.
Cover design by Heath D. Alberts

ISBN-13: 978-1523662920
ISBN-10: 1523662921

FIRST DIGITAL NINJAS MEDIA EDITION – Published In The United States – 01/23/16

16　17　18　19　20　21 ❖ 10　9　8　7　6　5　4　3　2　1

Original Works By Digital Ninjas Media

Fiction
Terminal Beginning
Last Rights
The Battery Man
Deeper
Photographic Memory
Not On The List
A Twist Of Fate
Rockford Writes (Contributor & Editor)
The Meaning Of Light

Non-fiction
Guerrilla Business
Guerrilla Business 2.0
Dave's Not Here

The DNM Historic Revival Collection

Fiction
The Sock Stories Omnibus
Tamerlane & Other Poems

Non-Fiction
Fasting For The Cure of Disease

WARNING & DISCLAIMER: While Dr. Hazzard may have begun her work with the best of intentions, it is clear to me that her actions took on a much more sinister tone throughout the course of her practice. She inflicted an inexcusable breach of trust and confidence upon her patients – some to the point of their ultimate and unnecessary demise.

This book is NOT to be used for medical purposes in any way, shape, or form. Ever. *Period.* I am not a doctor, nor does one sit on staff with the publisher. Before ANY medical action is considered, one should always consult a licensed physician. This holds doubly true for medical 'advice' – regardless of potential merit – that is found throughout this book.

This work is presented as a republication of a piece of insightful history which, the publisher felt, offered up further material for those who might be curious about Dr. Hazzard's doings. It dovetails nicely with television programs and films on the topic, as well as the excellent work, "*Starvation Heights*", by Mr. Gregg Olsen. I know this, because this is how I myself came to possess an original copy of the work. It sits in my collection right beside Mr. Olsen's book, as a sort of macabre compendium.

Once more, I urge you: do not treat this work as anything more than a historical insight. Always consult a physician with matters of personal health, and do NOT attempt anything contained within these pages. Ever. Unless instructed to do so – specifically - by the aforementioned physician.

Heath D. Alberts
Rockton, Illinois, January, 2016

FASTING FOR THE CURE OF DISEASE

BY
DR. LINDA BURFIELD HAZZARD

ORIGINALLY PUBLISHED BY

THE PHYSICAL CULTURE PUBLISING
COMPANY

NEW YORK CITY, U. S. A.

1908

CONTENTS

PREFACE - 15
I. FASTING - 17
II. STARVATION - 21
III. WHEN AND WHY TO FAST - 23
IV. PREPARATION FOR THE FAST - 29
V. SYMPTOMS - 33
VI. THE DURATION OF THE FAST - 45
VII. BREAKING THE FAST - 49
VIII. THE ENEMA - 53
IX. FOOD AND DISEASE - 59
X. REST AND ELIMINATION - 63
XI. AUXILIARIES IN FASTING - 67
XII. DIET - 73
XIII. MENTAL AND BODILY REACTION - 79
XIV. CHILDREN IN THE FAST - 85
XV. SEXUAL DISEASES AND THE FAST - 91
XVI. DIFFICULTIES IN CONDUCTING THE FAST - 95
XVII. CURES BY FASTING - 103
XVIII. DEATH IN THE FAST - 119
XIX. SCHOOLS OF NATURAL HEALING - 137
GLOSSARY - 141

PREFACE

The several years that have passed since the second edition of this work was issued have brought daily proof of the success of the claims then made. In this, the third edition, the author trusts that improved form, more numerous citations, and greater detail will serve to stimulate both the scientific and the popular mind to a realization of the importance of systematic investigation of the theory and the practice of Fasting for the Prevention and the Cure of Disease.

Again the author desires to acknowledge her indebtedness to Dr. Edward Hooker Dewey, now deceased, for his counsel and personal guidance in the early years of her practice. She is also deeply sensible of the encouragement and material support of patients and friends, in default of which the success that has attended her efforts in advancing the work in hand would many times have failed of accomplishment.

The author cannot flatter herself with the thought that she will succeed in convincing all who read this book of the truth it presents, for any question that concerns inducing belief in other minds is seldom settled by argument. But, if it be capable of practical solution, its worth is easily discovered through trial. And it is thus with the fast. But, because of almost universal dependence upon specialized advice, and because of human desire for tangible remedy, the method is hard to follow. It involves rigid self-denial in its initial stages and after it is broken it may prove disagreeable in application. If, for one moment, the immeasurable benefits that accrue from bodily purification and renewal are lost sight of, bitter lessons are taught. The slow processes of nature can never be hurried in action. Time elapses in the development of disease, and time must elapse ere cure results. Impatience is the evil underlying world-dependence upon drugs. Quickness of action is demanded, and a symptom suppressed is a cure accomplished in medical parlance. But, is this true? The text explains.

Every step that is taken in developing the practice of treatment of disease by natural methods is met with opposition which, in many instances, amounts to persecution. The research covered by this work, and especially that which involved post mortem examination, was hampered by medical intervention and was accomplished only through sheer determination and the assistance of a few broad minds in authority. The author believes that these autopsies are unique in the history of the healing art. No other investigator in her ken has had opportunity to connect the origin of disease with the immediate cause of death its organic consequence. The latter, in all cases, have the additional advantage and scientific value of being exhibited free from the effects of drugs.

Stress must be laid upon the truth in the statement that the fast is but a means to an end. Full vigor and complete recuperation are not to be had in a moment, and the completed benefits of the treatment are seldom enjoyed until three, four, or six months after the end of abstinence. Patience, self-denial, and faith are the moral requirements, with physical regeneration as the reward for their exercise.

In describing the symptoms of disease and the anatomy of the body, it has been necessary to use terms that are technical in character. To render the text perfectly intelligible to the lay mind, a glossary has been appended which contains the definitions of all words difficult of interpretation.

The facts presented and the arguments made are intended primarily for general intelligence; but, since the facts are corroborated, it is hoped that earnest investigation will follow by those who seek truth in its every phase. The author claims no originality in theory, either philosophical or physiological, but she insists upon the recognition of her thoroughness of detail in research, and of her confidence in practical demonstration.

LINDA BURFIELD HAZZARD
Olalla, Washington, December, 1912

CHAPTER I: FASTING

'Appetite is Craving; Hunger is Desire. Craving
is never satisfied; but Desire is relieved when Want is Supplied.
Eating without Hunger, or pandering to Appetite
at the expense of Digestion, makes Disease inevitable.
Some, as thou saws't, by violent stroke shall die,
By fire, flood, famine; by intemperance more
In meats and drinks, which on the Earth shall bring
Diseases dire, of which a monstrous crew
Before thee shall appear, that thou mays't know
What misery the inabstinence of Eve
Shall bring on men.
If thou well observe -
The rule of "Not too much" by temperance taught
In what thou eat'st and drink'st, seeking from thence
Due nourishment, not gluttonous delight.
Till many years over thy head return;
So may'st thou live, till, like ripe fruit, thou drop
Into thy mother's lap, or be with ease
Gathered, not harshly plucked, for death mature.'

John Milton, *'Paradise Lost'*

In order that a clear grasp of the subject matter of the text may be obtained, a short explanation of the fast and of the principles upon which its efficacy in the treatment of disease is based is essential. It will also be necessary, for the purpose of defining the distinction that exists between Fasting and Starvation, to discuss in a following chapter the physiological changes developed in the progress of the latter, since, in the popular mind, the two processes involved are vaguely considered as one and the same.

Fasting is defined as follows: The voluntary denial of food to a system, which is diseased, and which, because of disease, does not require nourishment until rested, cleansed, and eager again to take up the labor of digestion. Then, and not till then, is food supplied; then, and not till then, does starvation begin.

Relieving physical illness by voluntary withholding food is based upon the logical conclusion of the argument herein that, no matter what are the various names attached to the forms in which disease is manifested, there is but one cause for all of its outward and inward signs. The sole source of bodily ills is impure blood. The cause of impure blood is imperfect digestion.

An important distinction in conditions here needs exposition:

Organic disease, whether inherent or the result of continued functional disturbance or physical shock, is that in which one or more of the internal organs of the body is deformed, undeveloped, or otherwise disabled so as to prevent or to curtail its work, a state comparable to that of a machine with a missing cog.

Functional disease is that in which the organs themselves are in condition to do their work naturally, but have become unable to function because of poisonous congestion, the result of food taken into the body beyond the amount which the system needs for maintenance. Such surplus ferments and putrefies in the intestinal canal and elsewhere, producing toxins that are absorbed into the blood, thus impairing its quality and functionally hampering the vital processes. Extra labor is also entailed upon the organs assailed, since they are stimulated in unwonted degree by the presence of substances harmful to their action.

Inherent organic disease is a cause in itself of imperfect digestion, for, when it is present, the organs are partially or entirely crippled from birth. While this form of disease is beyond the hope of cure, its harmful results upon the body may be reduced to a minimum by means of the fast, and a combination of this method of treatment with scientific dieting will lengthen the life of the unfortunate victim to the extent to which a defective organism permits vitality to operate.

Functional disease and its ultimate result, functionally-caused organic disease, are the consequences of digestion impaired by incorrect methods in feeding, by improper selection of food, and by excess supply. In any of these circumstances, as has been said, poisons are produced that injure the system, until finally the condition becomes general and disease is apparent. As a matter of fact, the subject cannot have been ignorant of internal disturbance for some time previous to actual disability, for minor aches and pains have given ample warning. Mild preventive steps, taken when symptoms first appear, shut off by anticipative action later drastic measures. "An ounce of prevention is worth a pound of cure." The power resident in nature of contending against bodily abuse is limited only by individual characteristics, and a positive halt is not called until, through neglect, the physical machinery has been clogged with food rubbish and its products, and equilibrium has been overturned.

It is possible that at first sight the principles here set down cannot be fully apprehended, but, as important premises to the argument, they are again enumerated for reference by the student in connection with the body of the text:

The source of all symptoms of disease is impure blood.

Impure blood is caused by impaired digestion.

Impaired digestion results from

(a) Taking into the body food wrongly selected in kind or in quantity, wrongly prepared, or wrongly masticated.

(b) Taking into the body food that may have been correctly selected, prepared, and eaten, but in quantity greater than is needed for the repair and growth of tissue cells.

If any of these causes is operative, food ingested ferments and putrefies, generating a circulating poison that creates and continues disease until the producing cause can be cast out by the organs of elimination. Inherent organic disease and functionally-caused organic disease in its later stages embody defects in form, size, or cell-structure of any one of the vital organs. Except in rare instances, through surgical intervention, such structural deficiencies are beyond the hope of cure, but a scientific dietary, combined with judicious application of the fast and its accessories, will afford relief and prolong existence.

In purely functional disease the vital organs are normally developed and physically perfect in structure, but, clogged and laden with the accumulation of the toxic products of food excess, their functions are impeded or totally arrested. Functional disease is a condition that admits of complete recovery, and, even in its acute forms, cure is a certainty where natural law is permitted its course.

Any symptom of disease in the body is evidence of poison circulating in the blood and deposited in the tissues. The conventional medical method of attack invariably aims at the suppression of the symptom rather than at the removal of its cause.

Hunger and disease cannot exist simultaneously in the human frame, and natural methods of cure take this fact into consideration, assuming first, the unity of disease, and second, the means indicated by nature for restoration of health. When hunger is absent, food is not required, and all animate creation, save man, obeys the primal law of abstinence when the physical scale no longer balances. Recognizing that disease arises from a single source, the method of the fast recognizes as well a unity of cure rest for organs overworked and abused, and prompt removal by natural mechanical aids of filth productive of substances noxious to health.

To revert to the symptoms of disease the function of digestion is generally regarded as an extensive and complicated process, and it is so closely related to the functions of other parts of the body that it is difficult to describe the bounds, if any, beyond which digestion has no influence. The digestive apparatus is commonly spoken of as including the alimentary canal and those important glands that contribute secretions to the successive processes involved; but, as absorption and assimilation, on the one hand, and formation and withdrawal of waste products, on the other, are so nearly related to preliminary digestion, it is impossible to form a clear conception of disease of the digestive organs without observing the state of other and contributory parts of the body. While it makes for simplicity of description to exclude those organs not commonly grouped with the digestive apparatus, this does not result in a correct understanding, and therefore, if an explanation is to be found, not only for a disturbed physiological state, but also, in instances, for structural changes in the digestive organs, the field must be widened, and study be directed to the nervous system, including its physical manifestations, to the fluids of the body, to the rebuilding and breaking-down of tissue, and to the eliminative functions as well. Unconsciously, a great part of the importance of this general view is perhaps recognized when it is assumed that good digestion depends upon restful sleep, fresh air, sunlight, physical exercise, and activity of the bowels, kidneys, and skin. Disregarding these essential matters, it is difficult to apprehend the nature of digestive disturbances, or to prescribe for their relief. It may truly be said of an individual that, in a sense, his digestive ailment arises in the brain, in the lungs, in the heart, or in the kidneys, but the distinctions and differences heretofore stated must be clearly kept in mind, lest the idea of the unity of disease be clouded. The study of disease of the stomach is not limited to that organ, but is the expression there of disturbances that may be widely distributed throughout the body. Medicine has sought to give disease specifically classified names based upon locality of symptom, but this, it is seen, is only a relatively justifiable conception. There are no symptoms referable solely to the kidneys, to the heart, or to the blood; the man is sick from a single cause; his illness appears here or there.

The advance toward unity of thought and of action goes on in all scientific fields, and it is logical to believe that the important place occupied in the universe by the body of man should long since have been completely defined, and that the disturbances of the physical functions of the human edifice should have been traced to their single source.

The doctrine of Unity in the Cause and Cure of Disease, as set forth in the text of this work, has been carefully and earnestly investigated through a period of over sixteen years. Thousands of cases have been handled, and each instance has confirmed the conviction that the principle involved is absolutely sound. It has stood all tests. Where death has occurred, the autopsy showed organic defects, inherent, or acquired through years of continued functional abuse. These defects alone made death inevitable, whether the patient be fasting or feeding.

So far as can be accomplished in a work of this size, the fasting method of cure and the results of its application in the regeneration of the body and the mind are fully discussed. All that is asked of the reader is that prejudice be laid aside, and that the subject be approached without bias, keeping before the eye of the mind the words of the Apostle: "Prove all things; hold fast that which is good."

CHAPTER II: STARVATION

'Repletion and Starvation may both do harm in two contrary extremes.'

Burton, *'Anatomy of Melancholy'*

Death from starvation frequently occurs when the body is overfed. The purpose of food is that of nourishing body tissue, a purely mechanical process for use in growth and rebuilding. In the event that, through errors in digestion, organic defect, or fault in the functions of absorption and assimilation, tissue waste is not replaced as broken down, starvation and death result. If any one of these conditions exists, the more food supplied, the less resistance to disease succeeds, since energy is then directed towards the elimination of food products that cannot be utilized because of physical inability in the ultimate processes of growth. Exhaustion and, after a time, death occur.

Death from starvation cannot take place in a fast when organic disease is absent. In every animate body a reserve supply of nourishment is held in the interstices of tissue cells. The brain and the nerves are directly mine disasters, and the like, digestive function is paralyzed primarily by mental apprehension due to the situation. If death occur in these circumstances, within several days or weeks, it must be attributed, not to want of nourishment, but to the effect of general emotional exhaustion upon physical force.

For the purposes of the text, Starvation may be defined as the denial of food by accident or design to a system, non-diseased, but clamoring for sustenance. Hunger indicates the need, and, whenever its call is sounded, fatal consequences ensue in case of neglect or omission to feed.

Thus emphasizing the distinction between the state of the human body in a fast, and its condition in the process of starvation, detailed examination of these subjects is left for other chapters.

CHAPTER III: WHEN AND WHY TO FAST

'The When The Why It Boots It Now To Tell.'

Byron

It is, perhaps, difficult for the average mind to grasp the fundamental natural principle of the Unity of Disease to realize that disease is not only the warning of nature, but her remedy in sickness. The symptoms expressing disease may be specifically named and classified it may be said that a patient suffers from Bright's Disease, from eczema, from diphtheria, or from smallpox, but behind the symptom lies the cause, and the body is not to be thought of as ill in a special locality or in an individualized organ. It is sick as a whole, though the signs of its ailment are more visible or more severely expressed in one locality or another. Illness results when balance no longer exists between nutrition and elimination, with the consequence that the blood-current is vitiated at its source, the resistive powers lowered, and germ-soil produced. One remedy alone can cope with this condition, and it is that which nature suggests and employs elimination of the poisonous products of digestive ferment, and rest for organs, that have been functioning under stress. It is thus seen that, not only is a unity to be recognized in the cause of disease, but that there exists an equal unity in natural means of relief and cure.

Here is perceived the peculiar office of the fast it is the unit cure. As pointed out elsewhere, the lower animals by instinct employ it when ill, and its efficiency in disease, functional and organic, when applied to humankind, is fully substantiated and daily corroborated.

Disease affects every cell in the animal body. The fast in its operation and results equally affects the body as a whole. What matter, if, in attaining the extreme ends of purification, the body is reduced to a minimum of flesh? Organs and frame-work still remain by which and upon which to build a new, purified, and resistive structure for future needs.

The simplest forms in which bodily illness is expressed are the various rashes that appear upon the skin. These result directly from stomach-abuse from inability of that organ to carry on its work because of overwork or of food improperly supplied. Elimination through bowels, kidneys, and lungs is by nature continued to the limit of the power of these organs. They may be overtaxed, and then but one avenue remains for the escape of surplus impurity the skin. It responds, and in responding, suffers. Sometimes it is the skin itself that is called upon to work to its limit, or it may be that it is affected by exposure and chill with closing of its pores; then the excess of waste is discharged through mucus membrane or through lungs, and colds and pneumonia appear. Equal balance must exist among all the organs of elimination. Each must perform its allotted task proportionately with the others. And the arms of the scale of intake and outgo must likewise remain at level, and they do so maintain balance in health. Any excess of weight on one side or the other means disease. The fast as a remedy is universally indicated never specially so. There are no diseases, but only one disease. And for this there is but one remedy. No need exists in health for the employment of measures for the alleviation of pain and distress, for the reason that these signs are non-evident when physical balance exists. Remedial means are necessary only in illness, and then, and then alone, should the fast and its accessories be applied.

Before entering upon a fast, illness must be manifested, and the patient, whether under guidance or conducting his own case, should fully grasp the details of the truth that physical lack of balance is due to a single cause. The symptoms that are present, or that may arise thereafter in the fast or when on diet, need occasion no alarm, for their source is understood, and their meaning is a therapeutic one. Nature is in process of purifying the body is casting out its waste, and is cleansing the system in preparation for active, healthy rebuilding. The omission of food permits natural law to operate unhampered, and it is the only method by which natural assistance can be given with the assurance of permanent relief and cure. The alleviation of symptomatic distress is accomplished locally by simple hygienic means dry heat, hot fomentations, cold applications, sunlight, fresh air, osteopathic manipulation, chiropractic adjustment, and the enema.

The time to fast is when ill. And illness never occurs at the convenient moment. Its warnings may be present in summer or in winter, and they must promptly be heeded regardless of personal inclination or of climatic condition. To wait until disease develops locally is disastrous, and diagnosis is unnecessary, for natural treatment in any and all illness is identical in essence, and varies only in minor details. True, it is more pleasant to carry out a fast in warm weather, but this should never deter an ailing body from fasting in winter. Artificial means of maintaining room temperature are always available, and the hygienic requirements may be utilized with equal success whether the outer air be warm or cold.

As a matter of fact the substance of the argument indicates that winter is the natural season of rest and recuperation. Outdoor nature is dormant. Many animals hibernate, and all prepare for the growing period, the resurrection of spring. Mankind, because of artificial environment and custom, and with the mistaken idea that body-heat is derived entirely from fuel consumed, from food ingested, eats more heavily in winter, and approaches spring with a system overloaded with waste and in no condition to meet the work-time of the year. Spring-fever and spring-tonics are household terms, and epidemic disease is more prevalent then than at any other season. But again, remedy for disease should be used only when disease is manifested.

On the other hand, the social surroundings of a fasting patient are of the utmost import. The effect of mental states upon the physical body is too well known to dwell upon in this connection, and another chapter deals with this subject in all of its aspects. When friends and family object to the treatment, they object because of ignorance of the purpose of the method and of the details of its application. Affection, too, may enter into their opposition, and they, in their ignorance fear the outcome. The simple truth that underlies the method is usually easy to impress upon a mind situate in a body long diseased. But, often, convincing a patient is only half the battle, for relatives and friends resist to the point of compulsion. Since peace of mind and quiet environment are essential to successful issue, it is best to remove from anxious but misguided intimates, permitting them to await in ignorance of immediate trials the results that prove the wisdom of conviction.

Worry, anger, and grief are also most detrimental to progress towards cure. One instance comes to mind in which a case had fasted but eight days for functional disease of no especial gravity. Improvement had been continuous, but differences existed between the patient and her husband, and the latter, in an interview with his wife on the eighth day of her fast, so angered and distressed her that a nervous congestive chill, with suffusion of blood to the brain and lungs, occurred, and death resulted immediately from these causes. No amount of argument could convince the orthodox mind that the fast had not brought about death in this case. But the woman would have died just as surely had the scene described taken place before the omission of food, when the patient was ill and nervously weaker than at the time when anger and grief were so strongly excited.

In cases of functional disease, when the patient is not so depleted as to be bed-ridden, moderate daily exercise is most beneficial. In fact, it is recommended that the ordinary duties of life be continued, if such be possible. In many instances this can be done, and benefit accrues from exercise, because of its assistance to elimination, and from mental work, because of its value in diverting the mind from contemplation of physical ills. Numbers of fasters can safely follow their usual vocations, and, again, others are compelled to rest throughout the period of abstinence. The majority of the latter are, however, sufferers from organic defects, incipient or advanced in character, and sooner or later the facts are uncovered in the course of treatment.

One thought may be impressed at this point. The patient should so occupy himself, in so far as he can, that his illness and his treatment are not at any time uppermost in his mind. The method in its infancy has numbered among the majority of its patients chronic invalids, medically treated for years, and accustomed to constant thought of personal pain and distress. The relief occasioned by the fast very often permits these cases to forget their ailments, and to devote their attention to the duties of life. Occupation and amusement assist materially in accomplishing this result.

In the ordinary case of functional disease the fast to complete purification should be employed. The law of hunger determines its duration, and, all other things being equal, the surroundings and mental attitude in accord, this course will assure restoration to health. When the environment is not congenial, or when, in the mind of the director of treatment, the condition of the patient is such as to require the suggestive effect of food, occasions may arise when the partial fast or the interrupted fast may be used to advantage. Sometimes, too, the facilities for carrying out a complete fast are not at hand, and here the partial fast may be deemed a better policy than its finished product. The end is eventually identical, although it is somewhat longer in accomplishment when the partial or interrupted fast is employed.

There are cases in which the poisonous products of digestive putrefaction are present in such quantity as to tax the eliminative organs beyond their capability. In fact, when serious and extreme symptoms occur after the beginning of a fast, it is virtually certain that organic defects exist, and caution and knowledge are then needed in carrying the fast to its conclusion. Because of the general belief that every symptom is a separate disease, the ordinary mind regards the symptom to the exclusion of the disturbance producing it. When a symptom of disease appears in aggravated form after years of intermittent occurrence, experience leads to the conclusion that organic change has taken place, and that disease is due no longer to functional derangement, but to actual organic defect. Here the partial or the interrupted fast is found desirable, not because the protracted fast would not accomplish the results with better prospect of successful outcome, but because the average patient regards the symptom as the cause, and fails to appreciate what its temporary aggravation in the protracted fast implies. Increase in severity of symptom may occur and does occur in periods of dieting also.

An organ mechanically defective, especially if it be eliminative in function, cannot be expected to work to full capacity. It may be able partially to perform its task, but, pushed beyond a point, it will assuredly fail to respond. In the fast all vital parts are engaged in a supreme process of purification of casting out waste matter. And, when it is seen, through aggravated symptoms, that one or other of these is incapable of full duty, the progress of elimination may be checked by interrupting the periods of abstinence with intervals of diet.

The only alleviation that can be accomplished when distress occurs in a fast, is that which may be obtained by assisting nature hygienically. Little can be done in case of severe symptoms save to await results, but the enema is an all-important ally, and invariably brings immediate relief, while hot applications for pulse and temperature below normal, and cold applications for the opposite condition, are essential as well. The partial and the interrupted fast, whether indicated in the manner described or entered into from policy, are always beneficial.

The post mortem examinations cited in the text reveal the fact that it is impossible for one to die in the fast unless the vital organs are in such condition prior to entering abstinence that death is inevitable whether food is taken or not. Symptoms severe in character result, in the fast or out of it, from organs that are below normal in size or that are misplaced or defective in structure. And, when distressing conditions arise in the fast, the safer and the saner thing to do is to continue the omission of food to the point of purification, rather than to return to feeding or to resort to the partial fast. The process of elimination accomplishes but one thing the casting out of waste and to return to feeding puts extra labor upon organs already overtaxed. Vital parts are often defective in structure due to wrong treatment in the growing period, or to inherent deficiency, and then, when the fast is invoked, the symptoms are invariably distressing. When, during the omission of food, symptoms of pain and distress are aggravated, and resort to food is taken, the trouble is only increased, and the patient finds himself in deeper water than before.

Fruit juices and liquid vegetable foods are the proper diet indicated when the fast is broken before its completion or at its logical end, since these are easily handled and place no great tax upon digestion. When acid fruits are not tolerated, the fast may be broken on vegetable broths alone. Various vegetables and cereals lend themselves readily to the preparation of broths suitable for the purpose named. Tomatoes, carrots, asparagus, rice, and barley, and garden produce generally may be utilized. But nothing can quite take the place of the broth from tomatoes, for this vegetable, though slightly acid in composition, seems to satisfy both taste and nutrition at any and all times. Even in a fast, when serious symptoms are present, the broth from the tomato may be given for the relief of distress. The preparation of this vegetable may be referred to as a counterpart of that of the others, and it is here described. Two pounds of tomatoes are stewed with about two cups of water. The boiling should continue for approximately fifteen or twenty minutes, and the broth should be slightly seasoned, then strained so that no large solid particles enter the stomach. One cup of this product served hot often answers as a means of complete relief from pain, and it is the ideal food upon which to break a fast as well.

The drinking of water during a fast is not needful unless thirst is indicated. When the latter sensation makes demand, only sufficient water to satisfy it should be taken. The forcing of water upon the body when no desire exists taxes organs already burdened. Water should not be thrown into the stomach in gulps. It should be sipped, especially when fasting, for it then causes no shock to the system. Thirst is not always evident in a fast, since, when properly conducted, water is supplied to the body through absorption from the vehicle of the enema. The kidneys are flushed from this source, and the fluids of the tissues are maintained in the same manner. A knowledge of this fact will relieve the tortures of the shipwrecked mariner, for an enema of sea-water, in addition to its cleansing properties, will satisfy thirst.

CHAPTER IV: PREPARATION FOR THE FAST

'Do not think that what is hard for thee to master if impossible for man; but if a thing is possible and proper to man, deem it attainable by thee.'

Marcus Aurelius Antoninus

When disease appears in humankind, it is, as said before, not only a warning but a curative process. The disturbing element needs removal, the tired, abused organs need rest and repair. Instinctively real food desire, true hunger, disappears; in fact, for some time previous to actual disability, hunger has been absent. Appetite or stimulated demand for sustenance may, however, remain in evidence even after illness is manifest; but disease and hunger cannot exist at the same time within the human body.

Bodily functions are swift in their adaptability to circumstances, and bodily organs accommodate themselves and their labors even to abuse. Consequently, in a system accustomed to years of excess food supply, nature carries on existence in spite of handicap until accumulation and subsequent decomposition institute disease. Were the subject to recognize the fact that prevention of later evil lies entirely in his own hands, the greater part of physical suffering would be eradicated; but prevention compels personal denial in personal habit and enjoyment; and denial in these respects is the hardest of all virtues to inculcate and to practice.

The simplicity of the application of the fast constitutes its chief drawback. To the mind convinced on final argument of the efficacy of the method, nothing is more easy than to begin the omission of the daily ration, irrespective of the mental and physiological changes that are involved. Food stimulation, always an important factor in disease, asserts the power of habit over the body; and, even though the will of the patient has been brought to understand the futility of dependence upon artificial aids to health, as embodied in medicine and in methods akin to it, general knowledge is lacking concerning the proper means to pursue in order to overcome habit and to meet the physiological mutations that ensue when food is denied the body for the purpose of prevention or of cure.

The cultivation of a habit is a slow and insidious process, and so, in lesser degree, is its destruction. Abruptly to cease an act or a bodily function that has become constant causes both physical and mental disturbances. Witness, for instance, the attempts of a victim of tobacco, alcohol, or morphine to escape from the toils. Will power, the highest attribute of mind, alone can accomplish the result. In many cases the will required to begin the fast is present, and food might at once be denied were this the sole consideration. But, because natural physiological change is always gradual in fulfilment, similar approach to absolute cessation of function is not only desirable but imperative. The ideal way of effecting the readjustment of organic action, that is the consequence of lowering to zero the intake of food, is to diminish by degrees the amount ingested. To omit all food suddenly when approaching a fast sets the stomach clamoring for supply at the hours which habit has fixed, and the results of deprivation are then comparable to those experienced by the toper or the victim of drugs when drink or narcotic is denied. Nervous reaction is at once apparent and depression follows. Only in acute disease should abrupt entrance to the fast occur, and this solely because nature demands at this time prompt and strenuous measures.

Daily baths and enemata, mechanical accessories for the maintenance of cleanliness and aids to elimination, mark the commencement of the treatment; and these accompaniments, with the omission of the morning meal, mark the first stage of approach to the period of total abstinence from food. Omitting breakfast and lessening quantity at the other meals paves the way; and, in the ordinary case of functional disease, the gradual diminution of food supply should occupy an interim of not more than ten days or two weeks, after which the other meals should in succession be dropped. Thus the system is prepared without any noticeable change, save that of relief, for entire deprivation of food, for the absolute cessation of the function of digestion.

In the event that the omission of the morning meal occasions undue distress, as sometimes happens, ripe fruit in small quantity may be eaten at the usual hour. Caution requires that sweet fruit and acid fruit be not mixed at any one time. Soups made of vegetables gradually becoming lighter in food value should constitute the remaining meals, which are successively dropped until all food is denied. It is well to use the juices of fruit alone for the last few days before entering the fast.

In the ordinary patient the omission of breakfast, as suggested above, causes slight disturbances, such as dizziness, headache, or stomach pains. These are the results of habit-change. Later they disappear usually within three or four days and there are ordinarily no unpleasant symptoms when the other meals are omitted. In the no-breakfast period, elimination of digestive toxins begins to gain over their formation, and, as the patient gradually diminishes ingestion, the fact that the body is undergoing a cleansing process becomes most evident from the daily discharges in the enemata, and from the odor that emanates from the skin and the breath. These results make it apparent that years of overburdened digestive functions and of consequent imperfect nutrition have loaded the tissues with toxins, and that a complete cleansing of the system, with rest for the organs of digestion and a rearrangement in nature and manner of food supply, is necessary for regaining a physical balance. A fresh foundation must be constructed as the old is removed, and a change in internal condition must be effected by destroying the active cause of disease, and by renewing, through rest, the functions of those organs that have been long hampered in operation.

The most important of the organs connected with the digestive process is the liver. It stands at the portal of the circulation of the blood like a faithful sentry. It receives digested food products, as they are absorbed through the walls of the intestines, and it separates that which may be used for the rebuilding of tissue from that which is waste. Its products are thus, on the one hand, blood filled with nutriment, and, on the other, the peculiar secretion known as bile. The latter it stores in the gall bladder, whence it is supplied to the intestines as needed in the digestion of food. Nature is loath to cast out any material as useless, and the function of the liver by which constituents of the blood, otherwise useless, are utilized for further digestive operation in the form of bile, is one of the most striking instances of her economy.

When overworked by overfeeding or other abuse, the liver cannot perform its function of inspection successfully, and more or less of the poison retained, absorbed from fermenting refuse in the intestines, is carried into the circulation. Excess of bile is manifested, and with it the headache, the cold, or the bilious attack appears, all warnings of further disease.

The minute cells of the liver have individual work to perform in separating nutritive matter from waste; and, unless care be taken to furnish a food supply correct in proportion and quality, bile is secreted in amount larger than the system demands or requires, and is itself absorbed and reabsorbed, with additions from other sources, until congestion results, the circulation is vitiated, and the bowels are filled with bilious toxins that poison and re-poison indefinitely. All habits having a tendency to cause digestive disturbance, such as the use of tobacco or alcohol, careless eating and overeating, hinder the functioning of the liver. Any clogging or interference with its duties prevents the blood from receiving the benefit of its inspection, and an impure product is the result. All parts of the body will show distressing symptoms of fatigue and of exhaustion if the cells of the liver become diseased or useless through intemperate living or through ignorance of the specific duty belonging to it as an organ of the human machine. And this, of course, is true with reference to the functions of any other of the vital organs of the body; but so closely is the liver allied to the immediate work of digestion that the detailed description given of its labors is deemed essential to a full understanding of the method discussed herein.

As will be discovered, there are two distinct plans to be followed when the fast is used as a means for the relief and cure of disease. One of these requires the patient to continue the period of abstinence to its logical and complete conclusion, the return of hunger, and its duration is problematical. The other, of equal value in milder complaints than those for which the finish-fast is employed, makes use of shorter intervals of abstinence from food, alternating with periods of restricted diet. What has been written in this connection may then be qualified to the extent that, when short fasts of one or two days, or of a week, are undertaken for the relief of temporary indisposition or for the prevention of acute disease, no such extended preparation as is described is needful. For the long fast, the fast that cleanses the system to purity, preparation as outlined must be precedent. The short fast and the compulsory fast in acute disease alone may be abruptly begun.

The salutary caution is added that, when impending illness is apparent, several weeks or even months of preparatory diet will render the system amenable to the complete cleansing results of the absolute fast, and, barring organic defects, will preclude many unpleasant consequences in symptoms. The value of the enema or internal bath during both the period of preparation and the fast itself, as well as its employment in health, will later be fully discussed.

CHAPTER V: SYMPTOMS

'Every excess causes a defect; every defect, an excess. Every sweet hath its sour; every evil, its good. Every faculty which is a receiver of pleasure has an equal penalty put on its abuse. It is to answer for its moderation with its life.'

Ralph Waldo Emerson

Disease symptoms are the evidences of the conditions present within the body, and they indicate with more or less accuracy the degree of functional or of organic disturbance. In addition they enable the experienced observer to localize the point of least resistance, the organ prevented from proper performance of its task. In fasting, these signs of disease, during the first days of abstinence, are seen to be exaggerated or seemingly increased in severity; but this is a logical consequence of the application of a method, the purpose of which is that of elimination of a clogging, circulating poison. The extreme process of casting-out in progress during the fast uncovers the seat of disease, and exaggerates in the very cure itself its characteristic signs. To the orthodox mind this phenomenon at once suggests an increase in severity, since to it the symptom itself represents a cause. But, regarding disease as a unity, or as arising from a single primary source, the intellect trained in the application of natural means of treatment finds no cause for fear, but rather reason for rejoicing. Nature has entered the open avenue of assistance presented and is proceeding rapidly to effect relief and cure.

In any method for the treatment of disease nothing can be done unless nature co-operates. In some methods her means of cure, elimination, triumphs in spite of the treatment, and this is nowhere so fully displayed as in traditional orthodoxy, which is trained to look upon the symptom, or the appearance of disease, as its cause. As a result the efforts of medicine have been directed to check, to suppress, to turn into other channels, the sign manifested. The fact has been and is ignored that, thus turned aside and unremoved, disease is certain of return in redoubled force.

The whole of the human race has been educated for years along wrong curative lines. For instance, in orthodoxy if the heart action is high, a depressant drug is administered; if it is low, a stimulant is given. In either case reaction occurs, and the organ is less able to recuperate when the clogged channels of bodily energy finally are cleared sufficiently for function. This occurs when nature asserts herself, as she often does, in spite of the drug. When the sign of distress appears upon the surface of the skin, attempts are at once in order, not to remove the inward cause, but to eradicate the outward appearance, "to drive it in." Orthodoxy refuses to admit the unity of disease, and hence neglects to assist in the cleansing process of nature, which, recognizing the cause, ignores the symptom, or uses it solely as a guide. The thought and hope of the physician trained to heed the warnings of disease from a natural viewpoint is this that the organs of the body of his patient may prove equal to the work of elimination, and this they can accomplish only when they are structurally intact. In spite of the mildness or the severity of its manifestation, it is through bodily purification alone that disease can be cured.

Since the physiological changes involved in the application of fasting for the cure of disease need to be made gradually, the ideal method of approach to the period of abstinence is to prepare the system by a gradual lessening of the food supply; but, whether begun in this manner or without preparation, as is necessary in acute disease, the resultant symptoms are in general alike. When the intake of food is stopped, the stomach is naturally emptied and commences its enforced vacation. All of its energy as an organ is then applied to recuperation, to allaying with the assistance of a blood-current continually gaining in purity, inflammation that may be present in its structure, and to relieving congestion in veins and in glands. It will from time to time be disturbed in this work by its neighboring organ, the liver, which, during the fast, becomes solely an instrument of elimination, and discharges quantities of refuse into the alimentary canal. The secretion of the liver is always a waste product, but, even as such, it has its use as a digestive fluid in health. When the fast is in progress, however, this product of elimination is discharged into the intestines, and is nothing more than poisonous refuse excreted from tissue, blood, and organs, which must be at once removed from the body lest it be reabsorbed into the circulation.

When food is taken away, the bowels still proceed to collect the waste deposited in them by the blood and the liver; the kidneys, the lungs, and the skin continue the process of elimination; and the whole sewerage system of the body centers its entire energy in an effort to clear away the impurities stored within. The stomach rests, while the involuntary absorptive functions continue their work, even upon excreted tissue waste; and, lest harm result, the most expeditious mechanical means must be employed to remove this product from the digestive tract. The blood, following its mission, gathers the refuse from cell structure, and supplies for rebuilding purposes what it finds available. This it discovers in the reserve supply of nourishment naturally stored in the interstices of tissue. As the process of elimination or purification continues, waste grows less; the density of the blood is reduced gradually, as refuse diminishes in quantity; and the labor of the heart is thus progressively lightened.

Heart action is low in some cases of disease, and it is high in others. It is low when the blood is loaded with waste and is dense or thick in quality.

It is high when fermentation of refuse in the intestines occurs, with absorption of active poison into the circulation. But, whether high or low, poisonous products are present in the blood. A circulating poison acting upon the nerves that control the heart may develop irregularities that seem to show organic structural defect, and these are often so diagnosed. But, following the argument of the text, it is plain that, whatever the symptom, improvement in heart action must necessarily result in the fast when elimination becomes sufficiently advanced to remove the poisonous refuse that is the cause of disease. No fear need be entertained as to the ability of the heart to perform its functions during a fast, for the organ has less work to do as each day goes by, and it is served with the increased nerve power of a system gradually purifying.

When the fast is once begun, elimination asserts its predominance. Desire for food is in many cases replaced by disgust at the thought of it, and appetite is lacking until the fast is complete. The very odor of food, and even the perfume of flowers is to some patients nauseating. When this symptom is present in aggravated form, it is an almost certain indication of organic defect that may prove fatal. In this sign, however, in both functional and organic disease, there may be variations, due more or less to the time devoted to preliminaries; and several instances are of record in which neither appetite nor a semblance of it was present throughout the entire period of abstinence. Other cases have claimed the sensation of false hunger from the beginning to the end of the fast.

Another general symptom is discovered in the fact that the tongue, immediately upon the omission of food, dons, in ordinary cases, a thick yellowish-white coat, which it keeps until the impurities within the body are eliminated; and the clearing of its surface is one of the important signals that indicate a complete and successful fast. When the secretions of the body are acid in character, an apparently clean tongue may develop, and in this event strict interpretation of the symptom might lead to the inference that the system is cleansed and is ready for food. But here pulse and temperature give needed guidance, and the condition of the mucus membrane of the mouth, or cankers upon the tongue are warnings sufficient for the practiced mind. The coat deposited upon the tongue is one of the simplest visible signs of an extremely foul internal state, and of the fact that elimination is rapidly taking place. In health a clean tongue, as defined medically, is seldom in evidence with a full stomach. Ordinarily here, food stimulation dominates elimination, for a foul tongue is only an indication of the attempt of nature to cast out impurity from the system. Except as previously stated, a clean tongue is one of the unfailing signs of a complete and successful fast, and it may take months to accomplish.

Like the tongue, the breath becomes loaded with evidences of the internal condition, and its odor is most offensive for the greater part of the fasting period. This, too, is an indicator of the progress of the cleansing process which the body is undergoing, and the termination of the fast is heralded by its becoming odorless.

One of the products of fermentation within the body is known by the chemical name of acetone. There is no doubt that acetone, the result of the decomposition of organic matter, is present to greater or less degree in many cases undergoing the fast. It is not necessarily a product of the albumen of the food, but is more probably the result of the destruction of that part of the body albumen that has come from the breaking down of the tissue cells. In other words, the producing material has served its purpose as living cell growth. In cases treated medically its presence is regarded with dread, and at times when it appears, as it does, in anaesthetized subjects under the surgeon's knife, operations have been abandoned because of the fear of death while the paralysis of the anesthetic endures. Its presence in a patient undergoing the fast indicates functional derangement of more than ordinary gravity. In health there is no production of acetone, since discarded cell tissue is eliminated before fermentation can occur. Once food is denied and cell refuse is discharged into the channels of evacuation, acetone, when it is present, appears in all the excretions, and its characteristic ether-like odor is most pronounced. In fact in these instances one of the signs of the beginning of the end of the fast is found in the disappearance of acetone from urine, breath, and excreta. It is no longer formed, since the body is again in position to produce normal healthy cell structure balanced by normal elimination of waste.

In disease it is quite usual to observe unpleasant body odors. These are manifestations of an unclean interior, manifestations which nature seeks to remove through the organs of elimination, not the least of which is the skin. One experienced in the treatment of mental diseases becomes expert in distinguishing the marked odor attached to most lunatics. Even in the milder nervous derangements, such as hysteria, the odor of the body becomes distinctly changed, and is frequently noticed by the patient himself. Effluvium is present in many disease symptoms other than those of the mind and of the nerves witness, for instance, the distinct odor characteristic of tuberculosis of the lungs. In the fast the one function paramount is that of elimination; and due to this fact the body odor at this time is decidedly more noticeable than in ordinary disease when food is supplied. So true is this that the presence of a fasting patient in a closed room can at once be detected by one familiar with the treatment and its results.

In cases of acute disease and in what is known as bilious temperament, after the fast has begun, annoying symptoms may develop, dizziness on rising suddenly, spots before the eyes, and general malaise and weakness. But these signs are not found in every instance and cannot be established as guides. Some there are who may abstain from food for from thirty to forty days without any disagreeable symptoms save an offensive breath and coated tongue, while there are others in whom all the signs, thus far described, are in evidence in gradually diminishing intensity until the end of the fast.

The experience of the fast is often trying to those who, by high living and overfeeding, have given the liver work beyond its capacity. Bile, extracted from the circulation and stored in gall bladder and liver, is cast out in large quantities and floods the intestines to such degree that, often before it can be carried downward, the stomach finds itself a depository for the surplus, which fact is noted by nausea and vomiting. There is no absolute certainty of the appearance of this sign, but it is usually present in the subjects referred to. In extreme form this symptom indicates a liver in some stage of disintegration, and recovery is doubtful. However, in one known instance during a fast, vomiting of bile occurred for twenty-six days in succession, with later restoration to health.

For the reason that excessive vomiting of bile is a symptom that indicates the probability of organic disease of the liver or of the intestinal tract, in these cases caution is urged in the application of the protracted fast. The symptom is not to be regarded as alarming when the fluid raised is yellow or yellowish-green in hue, and when nausea occurs at infrequent intervals. But, if the color changes to a vivid green or, as it does in instances of acute organic derangement, to black, the case may be considered as most serious in character and of doubtful prognosis. When nausea is present during a fast, it is far better to aid elimination in ridding the stomach of its contents through the mouth than to permit them to remain with the certainty of partial reabsorption and re-toxication. If difficulty is found in raising the contents of the stomach, titillation of the palate with the end of the finger or with a feather will cause the convulsive muscular contraction necessary; and the drinking of warm water will ease the act of retching and, at the same time, will cleanse the walls of the stomach.

There are patients with livers organically diseased who undergo the fast without the appearance of bilious vomit. Observation in post mortem examinations leads to the conclusion that these subjects are invariably effected with some stage of a cirrhosed or hardened liver, and are outwardly of an emaciated or wiry type. On the other hand, those in whom excessive vomiting occurs during the fast are always inclined to obesity and at death display a liver disintegrated or softened. Of the two types the chances for recovery are greater with the latter.

Bile thrown into the stomach may produce, through irritation of its walls, spasmodic contraction of the diaphragm, i.e., hiccoughs. They may also occur as the result of other abnormal stimulation of the diaphragmatic nerve, and this happens frequently in cases of any affection of the liver or of the intestines. When merely functional disturbance causes this annoying symptom, it may quickly be relieved by vomiting or by the drinking of cold water; but, if it persists, it points to serious conditions, and in the later stages of disease, it is proof of organic defects beyond repair and heralds the approach of death.

In the earlier stages of the fast there will probably be fermentation and consequent formation of gas in the intestines, which may continue for days, depending upon the amount of solid material clinging to bowel walls, and also upon what may be termed the virulence of the bile and other waste deposited in the alimentary canal. The gas formed is often the cause of colicky pains, and is always a source of uncomfortable moments until removed. Manipulation of the abdomen together with hot water applications are of great assistance in this event, since they tend to reduce inflated intestines by stimulating peristalsis, and thus bring about the discharge of the gas. The enema is also of the utmost value in these circumstances and must be employed.

In all cases in the fast the evacuations from the bowels are strikingly similar. Floating in a brownish fluid that shades to black in color are old feces more or less abundant in quantity. The latter are present for many days, and are evidence of the former statement that overworked bowels do not fully discharge their contents even when regular in action.

The more usual indication of disease as it affects body temperature is fever, but it is quite frequently the case that in anemic subjects, shortly after the beginning of a fast, the temperature drops to a degree or so below normal. This is caused by the absence of food stimulation, for a fast never lowers temperature. The latter is always below register in instances of long-standing debility, and it is high in proportion to the severity of acute disease. The fast tends to restore temperature and pulse to normal, be they high or low at its inception. It is well to note that, while the average normal temperature of the body is 98 2-5 degrees, and the average normal pulse is about 72 beats to the minute, these figures are not to be regarded as normal for each and every individual. There are variations both above and below that are not to be considered as arising in every instance from disease. A case is cited in which temperature before the fast was habitually ninety-four degrees; in the fast apparently no change was made until the twentieth day, when an increase of one-half degree was noted; average normal of ninety-eight degrees was reached ten days later. Here undoubtedly disease was the cause of low register. Many cases have been observed in which temperature at the beginning of the fast was so low as not to admit of register upon the clinical thermometer, but invariably average normal was reached before the end of abstinence. When conditions of abnormally low temperature are present during the fast, hot applications along the spinal column, and hot tub-baths are the means to be employed to assist internal elimination in restoring body heat to normal. In any case temperature is merely a symptom of the conditions within, and, whether high or low, it denotes that there is in progress a fight for life that has scarce need to be suppressed. No thermometer is necessary to read the severity of disease, and, if pulse and temperature are above or below normal at the beginning of the fast, they will descend or ascend to natural register when disease disappears, or perhaps while some of its symptoms are still in evidence. The general conditions described in this paragraph in connection with temperature below normal occur in the cases of almost all fasters. These are aggravated in certain temperaments, more especially in those who suffer from the wasting forms of illness, such as hardening of the liver, and mal-assimilation.

When the fast is concluded and the body has been rebuilt, it is to be noted that a vegetarian diet insures a pulse and temperature with no apparent tendency to rise above individual normal. If the dietary change has been one from flesh to vegetable, the pulse may show reduction of several beats from its former average.

One word more concerning bodily temperature in the fast: Physiology asserts and observation proves that there can be no digestion in the absence of digestive juices, and that there is almost no secretion of the fluids when fever is present. Why, then, feed during high temperature? Without digestion there can be no nourishment, no up building of wasted tissue. Why add the burden of eliminating undigested material to the already great effort that nature is making to reduce over-stimulated heart action and abnormal body heat? The surest means to correct this condition is to withhold food, to remove the refuse, and to rest those organs that are functionally unable to cope with the labor forced upon them.

Depending upon the physical tendencies of the individual, after the beginning of the fast and during its early stages, many symptoms not specifically described in this chapter may develop. In some a rash upon the skin appears, and in others a cold with excessive nasal and bronchial discharge is the form in which the purifying process at work is displayed. But these and all other signs that occur at this time may be ascribed in part to the depression succeeding food stimulation, and in part to the exceedingly great elimination of waste that is in progress. The latter is, of course, responsible for the larger number of symptoms that appear here and hereafter in the fast. After the first indications vanish, in cases of purely functional disease, the patient discovers that his strength has apparently increased, and that he is, in most instances, able to attend without difficulty to ordinary labor and to approach it with brain marvelously clear. In other words, with the loss of stimulation due to food poison, disease decreases, and real strength is manifest. The patient is not less weak nor more strong than at any time during his previous diseased existence when living under stimulation. The fast has but uncovered the true state of affairs, and it has demonstrated that a sick man is not of necessity a weak man, for weakness is absence of strength due to systemic poison alone, and, in the early stages of illness, strength is only dormant. This seemingly paradoxical statement is explained by the fact that in disease all avenues for the passage of energy and vitality are so clogged by cumulative waste products as to be rendered almost useless for the expression of these forces.

The subject of food stimulation has not received the attention that it deserves in any system of therapeutics, for it is always an important factor in disease. After the body has become accustomed to a fixed food supply, whatever the quantity or the hours of ingestion, it strenuously rebels when denied. The system may be greatly overfed; it may be slowly poisoning itself through its own indiscretions; yet the omission of a meal sets the stomach clamoring. Given the usual quota, matters progress comparatively smoothly until the excess proves too heavy to be carried, or some minute organism finds soil in which to increase and multiply; then nature calls a halt and attempts correction by her only remedy, disease. Opportunity occurs when the accustomed impetus, food, is removed, but the patient is plunged into the depths. Stimulation, so long a habit, now seems necessary to counteract the symptoms produced by deprivation, and here mentality must be called to the rescue, and the will must be asserted in order to overcome the disposition and the desire to resume feeding.

The kidneys, the lungs, and the skin are the main avenues through which the liquids of the body carrying with them soluble impurity are eliminated. In the fast, when any of these means of escape are clogged and their functions impeded because of defect in structure in themselves or in the intestines, or because of excess of waste, the salivary glands excrete in quantity, and constant expectoration of viscous, foul-smelling spittle is symptomatic of the conditions described. This symptom abates and ceases as the functions are restored, and it may be much alleviated by hot baths and by sweat-inducing fomentations.

The headaches of the fast are invariably located in the frontal portion of the brain, and are coincident with the prior stage of abstinence, when the system is accommodating itself to the physiological change of habit then in progress. As elimination proceeds this symptom disappears, and, in functional disturbances, the brain experiences more rapid relief from pain and distress than do the other organs. Connected with headache, when organic defects exist, are visual spectra and flashes of light. A muscular tremor, accompanied with a rotary motion of the eyeball, or even with crossed eyes and faulty vision, sometimes appears in the graver forms of organic disease. This peculiar variation in symptom has been observed shortly before death in the fast, and in extreme form it would seem to indicate approaching dissolution.

At an early stage in the fast partial deafness with humming in the ears is apt to occur. When this happens, careful and constant syringing of the outer ear with warm water discloses an excessive quantity of wax, after the removal of which, the annoying symptoms vanish. The presence of this secretion in amount above normal indicates the extreme of elimination to which the body lends itself while digestion is suspended. Cases, which, before the fast, have suffered from semi-deafness, find the symptom much aggravated until mechanical removal of the clogging mass of wax is accomplished. Every avenue of escape is utilized by nature in the process of elimination in progress during the fast, and the ears perform their part in company with the eyes, the nose, the mouth, and the eliminative organs themselves.

At the end of a fast remarkable evidences of complete renewal of the old body are dis- played. The hair falls profusely; tartar deposits upon the teeth are shed; diseased spots in dental substance are sloughed; and extreme forms of pyorrhea, those affecting the bone of the teeth, are wholly corrected. Finger and toe nails are sometimes replaced from beneath with complete new growth, the old horny covering being forced from position and cast off. All these indications demonstrate not only renewal of secretion and of cell-structure, but purification as well. In the rebuilding period perfect replacement occurs.

Emaciation in the fast cannot properly be regarded as a symptom. It is the result of the elimination of toxic products, together with the loss occasioned by the use by brain and nerves of the reserve food-supply stored in tissue interstices. Diminution of weight due to the latter cause is, however, very slight in comparison with that arising from elimination. Wasting of the body is greater in cases where the organs are atrophied or cirrhosed than in other forms of disease, but the loss is less in these instances than in those of functional disease or of organic hypertrophy.

Delirium in disease is not necessarily an alarming symptom. A temporary condition of mental aberration apparent in confusion of thought, incoherency of speech, and, in some instances, unconsciousness, is characteristic of certain natures, whenever the body temperature rises above a fixed point. This is possibly an inherited tendency, for, on the other hand, there are many temperaments whose minds retain control in any and all forms of disease, when the brain itself is not the seat of disturbance. In the treatment of functional disease by the fast, it is rarely the case that delirium occurs, and, if it does, its appearance is due to extreme auto-intoxication from excessive waste thrown into the intestines and not evacuated with sufficient rapidity. If present at all, it will be evident within a day or so after the fast begins, and it will cease when elimination has proceeded to the point of clearing the bowels from the congested mass of old feces. This symptom need never appear in cases of purely functional derangement, if proper preparation for the fast has been observed. In instances where abstinence from food is forced and involuntary, as is the case in mine accidents and in shipwrecks, the mental strain produced by the situation causes delirium, which, together with speedily fatal results, might be obviated were knowledge of the resources of the human body more general. In organic dis- ease, in the fast or before it, delirium may continue for some time, and, while its primary cause is one with that in functional troubles, its persistence is due to defects in organs that prevent elimination into the intestines, or to defects in the intestines themselves that hinder evacuation naturally or by mechanical means. If recovery be possible, these cases are most obstinate in yielding to treatment, for the process of cleansing is extremely slow and lengthy in accomplishment, while recuperation is delayed indefinitely. This class of cases requires more patience and caution than all others combined, since the patient is apt to become discouraged and to lose faith in. the power of nature to overcome the condition. Resort to food and drugs may again be had, and the outcome, doubtful before, is now inevitably fatal. The lesson to be learned when this situation confronts physician and patient is that of organic limitation. The vital organs are capable of function only within bounds, beyond which, are danger and possible death. Safety rests in natural processes alone; danger lies in tonics and in food.

A general classification of the symptoms of disease tending to limit certain signs to certain ailments can never be made with accuracy. It is true that medicine has ticketed and shelved all symptoms, and that it is its plan to await development of indications before diagnosis. But medicine devotes its attention entirely to the suppression of the manifestation to the neglect of its cause, and a classification thus made finds items overlapping each other in such manner as to make distinction difficult if not impossible. But an arrangement of general disease forms may be made on lines that are sharply defined.

1. Purely functional ailments that readily yield to the fast. In these cases because of accumulation of excess-food-rubbish in the digestive tract, blood, and tissue, organs are hampered in function but are not structurally defective or in themselves diseased. Gradual improvement is noted from the beginning of preparation for the fast, and recovery is always possible.

2. Organic defect in slight degree, occasioning disturbance because of work imperfectly performed by a partially disabled organ. This condition places heavier burdens upon other organs and functionally unbalances the entire system. Disagreeable symptoms are noted in these cases during the progress of the fast, and it is possible that full functioning may never be restored. However, if the structural defect has not reached the point that includes the case in the following class, and, if care be exercised during the period of convalescence, recovery is certain.

3. Organic defect of such degree that the functioning of a vital organ is

rendered impossible. A gradual decline, beginning before treatment and continuing with a short interval of relief after entering the fast, is the characteristic indication. The relief noted may be such as to offer hope of recovery, but, if the condition is as stated, there is no possibility of cure.

In functional disease, when her laws are obeyed, nature never fails of cure. She is helpless only when organic defects exist that defy repair.

The careful study of the symptoms of disease, as they occur either while feeding or fasting is in progress, reveals the law through which nature works to a cure. It may briefly be stated as a process of elimination, upon lines of least resistance, of the toxins produced by functions imperfectly performed. These signs of distress may often be locally relieved by mechanical means embodying heat, water, sunlight, air, and manipulation, but disease can never be eradicated by mere suppression of symptom. It must be removed at its source; and, despite its varied expression, there is but one cause, impaired digestion, and one remedy, elimination of resulting poison.

CHAPTER VI: THE DURATION OF THE FAST

'Physic, quick to affect the body, can never produce the perfect results of the slow operations of exercise and temperance the two great instruments of health.'

Addison

The duration of the complete fast is a matter that can neither be foretold nor prescribed in any individual case, for the treatment has its beginning in disease and its end in the hunger that marks the return of digestive power. Until the latter makes itself apparent, and it cannot be mistaken, the fast should continue. Then, and not till then, is the system in condition again to receive and transform food into tissue structure.

The sensation of hunger is a safeguard established by nature to insure bodily maintenance. It is the first instinct that the infant exercises at birth, and its office in all life is that of a watchful caretaker entrusted with interests beyond the ordinary in value. The natural consciousness of hunger has, in most individual instances, been usurped by artificial craving produced through the cultivation of the sense of taste and through regularity in the habits of feeding. Hunger is an involuntary function of the system as much so as is the beating of the heart. It is not created by the individual, nor does it make its appearance at stated hours by exercise of the will. But appetite, its counterfeit, is easily called into being and may be made apparent at set times.

In diseased conditions hunger is absent; and, in the fast, appetite ordinarily disappears after the first few days. When the elimination of toxic products is complete, hunger, not appetite, returns. Hunger is normal, appetite abnormal. This distinction with a difference is most important considered in connection with the breaking of a fast. The question of the resumption of feeding does not lie for answer in the hands of either physician or patient. It rests with the law of hunger alone. During the fast and until hunger returns, food of any kind is an intruder, and all of the energy of the body is being directed through the organs of elimination towards the cleansing of the system from its self-manufactured poison. The coated tongue, the foul breath, are simple signs of the decomposition of excess food and of worn-out tissue. And, being signs of decomposition, they are also signs of the death of life substance and of living organism, the products of which are harmful unless removed from the functioning body. When the elimination of these toxins has reached the point that rebuilding is demanded lest the body die, hunger will manifest itself. Hunger is the abiding law of animal existence; it is not a creation of man nor of the animal, but is the signal of instinct by which all animate creatures know that food is needed for the repair and growth of the organism. And, with its manifestation, the clean tongue, the sweet breath, and normal life symptoms return.

In functional disease the fast may be carried to its logical end without a particle of anxiety, for the law of hunger marks the limit beyond which abstinence cannot continue lest death occur. And to this nature has added another safeguard, almost its equal in importance. Resident in the body there exists at all times a supply of tissue pabulum for use in repair and growth, both ordinary and extraordinary. This is constantly called upon for the nourishment and up-building of nerves and brain, and the latter never suffer deterioration in substance nor in structure unless they themselves are organically diseased. Even in instances of death from alleged starvation, nerve tissue shows no loss. It makes use of the normal food reserve stored in the interstices of muscular tissue, and; fasting or feeding, it draws upon this accumulation for support. The whole nervous system regains its energy by rest alone, but it maintains its substance at par by the means described. Hence, so long as there remain tissue and blood sufficient to carry on the work of the functions and of the circulation, brain and nerves must continue their directing task, and they cannot waste in the process.

The statement, that a supply of healthy tissue-food exists during a fast and is not exhausted until natural hunger returns, does not rest for proof upon the mere assertion of medical observation in alleged starvation. In the chapter of the text devoted to cases cured by fasting an instance is cited of healing by first intention during a fast of fifty-eight days of a sore three inches in diameter, so virulent in character that the periosteum of the sacrum was exposed. Two cases of pregnancy are also noted in which the mothers fasted twenty-two and thirty days respectively. In the bodies of each of these women the growth of the fetus was progressive and normal, despite the total omission of food intake. Due to disease, hunger was absent in the pregnant women, but a supply of nourishment sufficient to maintain the body of the mother and to build that of the forming child existed within and was utilized until natural hunger returned at the completion of the fast. This stored nourishment is always present in tissue structure; it is the factor of safety in physical economy, and it is eliminated only at the time when in the fast complete purification of the system has occurred and hunger is asserted.

The signs of a fully completed fast are most easily recognized. The tongue is pink and clean, the breath, sweet, and appetite or false hunger is replaced by natural desire for food, a sensation exquisite beyond description, that may be realized only by a clean, pure, regenerated system. Natural hunger relishes natural food, and, once it is known, no morsel is without delight.

If the human body ate only when hunger makes demand, perfect balance would at once be created between intake and outgo, up-building and waste. Mastication, which is the mechanical part of ingestion, must, of course, be correctly accomplished to insure this result. Hunger is discriminative and preserves the body. Appetite is abnormal desire and ultimately destroys. Hunger is primarily indicated in the mouth, and, if not relieved, becomes an organic craving that can be satisfied only by digestible food; but appetite is silenced when even indigestible substances are ingested.

After the fast, with the return of normal hunger, the food selective sensations of taste and smell are also restored. These faculties in average existence are trained to accept material and odor abhorrent to naturally constituted organisms; but in normal state, while dependent upon true hunger, they act as minor indicators in determining the point that marks the conclusion of the fast. And with them thirst appears not that desire for liquid produced by stimulation or by drug-exhaustion of the fluids of the body, but that which makes known the immediate need for their renewal. The body that eats when hunger, not appetite, calls, that drinks when thirst, not stimulation, demands, and that follows unquestioningly the selective sensations of taste and of smell, need never know disease.

It is sometimes the policy of good judgment to break the fast before the system is completely cleansed, to return to it after an interval of dieting; but this is so, solely because of the wide-spread ignorance of the human body and its care, and because of the advantage that orthodoxy has taken of this fact for commercial and other reasons. The mind of the patient thus becomes imbued with groundless fear of death, and more harm than good results on account of the mental strain. From the same motive, policy may indicate shortening the period of abstinence when the certainty of the presence of organic disease exists, or when preparation has been carelessly performed or entirely omitted. But, even though organic defects are present, the body in disease is more certain of recovery when the fast is applied, since the labor of the organs is in process of gradual reduction, and progressive relief is afforded the system as a whole. The only hope of partial recuperation or of permanent cure lies in the rest given to overworked or defective organs, permitting them, if possible, to recover and to resume their functions.

The question regarding the duration of a fast is, then, one that can never be answered with certainty, and it is to be remembered that each individual develops his own case, and that each case has its own limitations and requirements. In view of these conditions, the fact is to be faced that no matured human body, in which disease is manifest, can be brought to health within a limited period of time. It has required years of abuse and of drugging to cause disease, and it is unreasonable to assume that nature in a few short weeks or months can bring about the physiological changes necessary to perfect functioning.

The fast completed, the body exists in a sphere of natural condition, and there are no circumstances in which there is so much of real gratification in the simpler acts that constitute physical life. To eat rationally, to eat only at the demand of hunger and not to excess, become exquisite pleasures, marred with no grief for the flesh pots nor for the loss of appetite.

What the fast requires is ability to follow logically the details of a great but simple law, the law of hunger, which, once obeyed, brings health for the asking, and demands only individual reason, effort, and will; but, once violated, condemns the offender to condign and lasting punishment.

CHAPTER VII: BREAKING THE FAST

"Tis in ourselves that we are thus and thus. Our bodies are gardens; to which our wills are gardeners: so that if we will plant nettles or sow lettuce, set hyssop and weed up thyme, supply it with one gender of herbs or distract it with many, either to have it sterile with idleness or manured with industry, why, the power and corrigible authority of this lies in our wills. If the balance of our lives has not one scale of reason to poise another of sensuality, the blood and business of our natures would conduct us to most preposterous conclusions: but we have reason to cool our raging motions, our carnal stings, our unbitted lusts.'

Shakespeare, *'Othello'*

Injudicious fasting, fasting without preparation, fasting for extended periods without guidance, and fasting for the sake of following a method merely because it is popular for the moment, are all severely condemned. The fast should be undertaken only for the cure of disease, and it should be scientifically applied. In disease, if adverse conditions, other than those apparent, are latent in the system, if nature has been carrying the burden of an imperfect organism, the fast is certain to uncover the fact, and symptoms will be revealed that need to be coped with by competent hands. It is, however, probable that, when purely functional derangements are in question, the self-guided patient will progress to a favorable end, but will not be equal to the problem of breaking the fast with success. This is a point of such importance that detailed comment is essential for the purpose of obtaining a clear insight into the matter of diet, hygienic care, and exercise after abstinence is ended.

An experienced director of the method is only too well aware that there are subjects, whose number entitles them to be distinguished as a class, who, through physical defect, store within the system extraordinarily excessive accumulations of food poison. These cases are grouped under Class 2 in the division of general disease symptoms noted in a previous chapter. In them constant stimulation prevents recognition of the presence of toxic products until some serious indiscretion overturns the balance, and a fast is begun, usually without preparation or direction. Once elimination has commenced, no return is possible until the logical end of the cleansing process is reached, and often alarming symptoms develop ere the first week has elapsed. The attempt is made at once to supply nourishment, and digestive trouble more severe in kind is produced, for the alimentary canal is filled with the products of elimination, and food but adds fuel to the combustion in progress. Fear now takes possession of the family and, more often than not, of the patient as well, and the deadliest foe to nature and her methods of cure is called to aid in offsetting the work already accomplished. Medicine completes in these circumstances what food began, and the chances are that death will ensue. No defense of the fast can be made, and it is visited with wide-spread and emphatic condemnation, whereas, were the facts known for their real worth, the conditions arising therefrom would be recognized as natural in origin, and as warnings that prodigious and successful efforts towards cure were at work.

To break the fast at a wrong time is even worse than to break it upon erroneous diet. The point of greatest import here to be observed is the care that should be given and the confidence that should be engendered lest fear step in and with it food and drugs. In the administration of copious enemata, duplicated and reduplicated, for the purpose of the immediate removal of disturbing elements lies the remedy for the eradication of alarming signs.

The fast in ordinary cases should be broken by the ingestion of the juices of ripe fruit, and of broths prepared from vegetables. The juices of perfectly ripened fruit are most easily changed in mouth and stomach for the subsequent process of assimilation. There is therefore but small effort in digestion. The same reasoning is applicable to the administration of strained vegetable broths seasoned to taste and void of solid particles. The thought that bids for this consideration of the digestive organs finds origin in the fact that the stomach has been for a time deprived of the exercise of its function, and return to solid food must be carefully made. The hunger instinct should guide, and, after all but a small amount of sustenance is needed to maintain the body. A caution is appended to the effect that the juices of sweet fruits should not be mixed at any time with those of acid. Vegetables in solid form and green salads are gradually added to the dietary as digestive power asserts itself.

There are many vegetables that lend themselves readily to the preparation of the broths referred to, and among them may be mentioned as particularly easy of digestion, ripe tomatoes, celery, carrots, and green peas.

Some of the cereals, such as rice and barley, are also easy to prepare and to assimilate in the form of broth. Great caution is essential in order to suit the diet to individual requirement, and slight experiment may be found necessary for a satisfactory solution of the problem presented.

In the infant, when hunger returns after the fast, the strained juice of stewed ripe tomatoes or of boiled carrots, both unseasoned, is most suitable preparatory food. To the carrots may gradually be added in small quantity top-milk and honey, but these should never be combined with tomatoes or with acid fruits. This regimen should be continued, varying the vegetables from which the broths are made and increasing their quantity as digestion advances, until the final teeth have been cut, and solids may be handled.

In late popular discussions of the treatment of disease by fasting and its accessories, patients have been advised to break the fast upon large quantities of cow's milk. From a chemical standpoint the milk of the cow contains all the nutritive compounds required by a growing animal, and contains them in the proportions of a correct scientific dietary. It does not, however, fulfil the conditions of a typical and model food when considered as sustenance for man. The chemical composition of milk renders it a most suitable soil for the cultivation of bacteria, and, even though pasteurized or sterilized, it will again take up germs if exposed to the air. In addition, sterilized milk is a different article from fresh milk, its chemical composition being altered by the process. The milk of the cow, when ingested, is changed upon encountering the gastric juices, into whey, a liquid, and into a tough mass of curd most difficult of digestion. To call milk a liquid food is absurd, for the solid matter in a pint of milk is equal to that in a half pound of meat, and in its dense coagulated form it is vastly more difficult of digestion.

In the present discussion the digestive capability under contemplation is that of an individual who has just succeeded in ridding his system of the toxic products of food in excess of the needs of the body. Hunger has returned and feeding must be resumed. If the milk of the cow is the form in which nourishment is supplied, and if, in addition, not one pint, but, as recommended, several quarts daily are imbibed, for each quart consumed, an equivalent in flesh food of one pound is offered for digestion. The purpose of the fast is at once defeated, since the most vigorous of bodies is unable perfectly to transform and to assimilate this mass of material. All of the excess and most of it is excess fills the alimentary tract with decomposing rubbish, and the system is again in the developing process of disease. A diet including ordinary quantities of milk succeeds at any time in depositing adipose tissue and in creating increased bilious flow. At the very best the milk of the cow is intended only as food for the calf.

When, after the fast, digestive power reasserts itself, the enemata are discontinued daily, but they should be administered without question at least twice weekly in health. That natural movements of the bowels are dependent upon perfect digestion is but slightly qualified by the statement that muscular tone is a necessary condition in the intestinal walls. For the attainment of this state, and for the rebuilding of general muscular quality, a system of judicious exercise is recommended and insisted upon when the fast is broken and thereafter. This, like diet, must be entered upon in gradual manner and is increased and extended in proportion as the body shows progressive capability.

The process involved in breaking the fast demands extreme caution and care. At the end of the period of abstinence and with the return of hunger, weak-willed patients are almost certain to overstep the bounds of supply. In these cases acute symptoms may develop, due to congestion of the entire circulatory system. The brain may suffer to the extent of the production of violent delirium, and all the organs of the body are included in the revolt. When a gradual process of return to normal amount in sustenance is not pursued, all the benefits of the fast are worse than destroyed, and, if will-power be lacking in the patient, its equivalent in supervision must be furnished by the director of treatment. If necessary, personal watch must be established over the convalescing subject.

When organic defects are present in the colon, they may or may not prove seriously shortening to life; but, when, at the end of a fast, feeding is resumed, even a slight displacement of the lower bowel may retard elimination to such degree that absorption of fecal material proceeds so rapidly as to cause severe physical and mental derangement. This is especially so in cases that are not under guidance, in which ignorance of consequence exists, and will-control is absent. Yet, even under competent supervision, oftentimes desire impels the patient to overeat.

This tendency must be controlled, for serious and disastrous results wait on premature excessive demand upon the eliminative function. Defective or normal in vital parts, man here learns to live within the limitations of his organs. The several portions of the treatment in comparison show the fast itself is easy of accomplishment. Resumption of feeding calls for greatest care.

CHAPTER VIII: THE ENEMA

'I keep as delicate around the bowels as around the head and heart; Divine am I inside and out.'

Walt Whitman

In fasting for the cure of disease, the enema is a necessary daily adjunct, and, while the fast is in progress, it should be taken on rising and before retiring. In health its use is advised at least bi-weekly, when it will be found a most relieving as well as cleansing operation, at once preventing accumulation and subsequent absorption of waste. In the event that it is administered directly after a movement of the bowels, convincing proof invariably follows that complete evacuation of the intestinal contents has not occurred; that there is a residue which, if not removed, will remain to ferment and putrefy. The necessity of this artificial aid to natural bowel movement is thus apparent. At the beginning of the fast, peristaltic action, in the absence of fresh supplies of food, becomes sluggish, and absorption proceeds through the walls of the intestines irrespective of the material present. The fluid state of the waste thrown into the bowels when the process of digestion is suspended, permits of easy absorption and of consequent septic poisoning. During the fast, from the first day of abstinence until indications point to the fact that the cleansing process is complete, large amounts of brownish foul-smelling discharges are evacuated, mixed with lumps of hardened fecal matter, dislodged from the walls of the intestines or impacted from particles excreted in the process of elimination. In long fasts another feature more or less noticeable is the quantity of stringy white or yellowish mucus that is evacuated. The latter is catarrhal in nature and is evidence of the complete renewal that is accomplished when the fast is carried to its logical conclusion.

The necessity for the use of the enema would cease to exist were all food ingested perfectly transformed and entirely consumed in tissue-building. But continued excess in supply creates imperfect functioning of the digestive organs. Natural bowel movements depend upon food perfectly digested or chemically changed, and the waste products from this process are always fully eliminated. Imperfect digestion causes imperfect elimination, which is the one source of septic poisoning and of subsequent disease; but so long as food ingested is cooked food and soft food, and so long as it is not properly masticated, just so long will assistance be required to evacuate the contents of the bowels. Inferentially this fact has been recognized for ages, since drug statistics show that ninety per cent, of all medication is aimed at the intestines.

Objections are made to the use of the enema on the grounds that it is not natural; that it tends to dilate permanently the bowel; and that its constant employment will ultimately destroy the functioning of the colon. In answer to the first difference it is found that drugs taken into the system for the purpose of causing a movement of the bowels pass through a process similar to that to which ingested food is subjected. They are acted upon by the digestive juices in the stomach and small intestine, and are absorbed into the circulation. The liver, in its capacity of separator, objects to their introduction as harmful to the system and casts out with increased secretion of bile that portion which reaches it. The nerves governing the absorptive and secretive functions of the stomach and intestines, irritated by the presence of a substance foreign and noxious to the digestive process, are stimulated into action and cause an augmented quantity of secretion to be poured forth, and the folds of the colon are filled with fluid fouled by dissolved fecal matter, which is partially absorbed ere evacuation can occur.

Purgatives in medicine are drugs which act as described, and they are divided according to their supposed peculiar properties. Thus there are cholagogues, that increase the flow of bile, and intestinal purgatives, that act on the intestinal secretion, e. g., calomel; or that increase peristaltic action, e. g., aloes and cascara. Again there are drastic purgatives or cathartics, e. g., croton oil; and mild aperients, e.g., compound licorice powder and senna.

Each application of the remedy finds the alimentary tract less able to contend against its presence, and, in order to obtain the desired effect in future, larger doses are necessary, more of the digestive fluids of the body are wasted, and the cathartic habit becomes as dangerous as continued indulgence in morphine. By it digestive juices are drawn upon to excess, digestion is rendered difficult, if not impossible, and constipation, with danger of septic poisoning, is aggravated. If the taking of purgatives were confined solely to adult life, the tale to be told would be utterly different in character, since functional derangement would be the principal harm effected. But cathartics are prescribed in infancy, and their indiscriminate use at this period of life is one of the great causes of intestinal mechanical defect, such as is described in detail in the chapter dealing with death in the fast. By their employment in childhood nutrition is lowered through resulting digestive disturbance; inflammation thus engendered is soothed with opiates; feeding and fermentation continue; development of the intestinal tract is arrested, or the tract in portions is functionally paralyzed an organic condition that cannot be corrected, even by nature itself, in a lifetime of later natural existence. How different the outcome were the enema administered in infancy when functional digestive disturbance and constipation occur! The results are immediate and are attained with no tax upon digestion. The delicate nervous fabric of the child suffers no disastrous reaction when bowel accumulation is thus naturally removed, and internal purity, the condition of health, is reached and thereafter assured.

To the objections that the bowel is permanently dilated, and its functioning lost by continued use of the enema, a detailed reply is necessary. The intestine, as a whole, is that part of the alimentary canal, which, commencing at the pyloric opening of the stomach, is coiled in the abdominal cavity and ends at the anus. For purposes of description it is divided into several portions. Food leaving the stomach passes first into the duodenum, then into the jejunum, and next into the ileum. These three sections form the small intestine, which in man is about twenty feet in length, but is subject to great variations. The lumen of the small intestine is larger at its upper end and gradually narrows as it goes downward. The opening of the ileum into the caecum, the first portion of the colon, is valvular, and this arrangement prevents any passage backward of the intestinal contents. Beyond the ileo caecal valve the caecum forms a large dilatation, and from it springs an elongated blind process, the vermiform appendix. The caecum is continued upward as the colon, which is described as (1) ascending, (2) transverse, (3) descending. The sigmoid flexure, a device of nature that prevents excessive pressure by the contents of the bowel upon the muscles of the rectum and the anus, lies between the descending colon and the rectum, whose lower opening, the anus, is guarded by a strong circular muscle. The sigmoid flexure thus interrupts the straight fall from the transverse portion of the large intestine to the rectum and acts as a retaining pouch.

From this description it will be seen that there are three positions in which the colon may receive a supply of water sufficient to soften its contents and to wash them away from its walls. These are the right-side, the knee-chest, and the flat-on-the-back. The latter, except in bed-ridden cases and in children, is inconvenient to assume, but the two former postures are found to be comfortable and easily taken.

When the patient in taking the injection lies on the left side, gravity can assist the flow only as far as the transverse colon, which in this position is a perpendicular tube forbidding further passage of the fluid of the enema. Hence only one-third of the bowel is possible of flushing. The right-side posture permits the water to flow along the descending colon, down the transverse bowel, and through the ascending gut to the caecum, completely flushing the organ. The knee-chest and the flat-on-the-back positions insure, with even greater ease, full cleansing of the bowel. When the injection is taken in the sitting posture, gravity and the contents of the lower portion of the bowel prevent the rise of the water unless some special device embodying force is utilized; even then only the descending colon receives the benefit of the flow, and dilatation of the rectum and the flexure is certain to occur, with possible mechanical injury.

Soap-suds, salt, soda, and the like are to be avoided in the preparation of the fluid in the injection. Similarly, oils of any kind are forbidden, and water warmed to body temperature, not higher than 100 degrees Fahrenheit, should be the only flushing agent. Absorption of a portion of the contents of each bag is almost instantaneous, so the safer plan lies in using no foreign substance whatever. Copious discharge from the bladder immediately after rectal injection is the common indication of the rapidity with which absorption occurs through the walls of the colon, and this, in itself, is proof that there is fallacy in the medical sub-argument against the use of the enema to the effect that no absorption of retained fecal material can take place. But medicine goes even further in the process of self-stultification when it recommends the employment of nutrient enemata. Denying that the contents of the bowels may be returned in part to the circulation through the walls of the gut, it nevertheless affirms that food material may in this manner be absorbed. It therefore assumes that tissue is nourished by matter that has not undergone the process of digestion. It is also readily seen that food absorbed through the walls of the colon is not received by the portal or nourishing part of the circulation, but enters directly into the venous blood, which is itself loaded with impurity awaiting elimination. To deliver household water to the faucets from the sewers of a city would be deemed an act of insanity, yet analogy is plainly evident when this method of transmission is compared with that of food introduced into the human body per rectum. When the patient is bed-ridden or abnormally weakened, the knee-chest posture in taking the enema may prove too exhausting; and, when this condition exists, a canvas stretcher upon which the subject may comfortably lie, can be placed over the bath tub. If this apparatus cannot be procured, a triangular platform of three boards covered with a blanket and oil-cloth, its base arranged so as to cross the top of the tub beneath the buttocks, may be used as a substitute. By this means all effort on the part of the patient in retaining position is removed, a matter of the utmost importance when excessive weakness is present.

The operator in administering the enema, or the patient himself, will often find it needful to repeat its application to the extent of twenty or more quarts, or until the fluid returns comparatively colorless. Observation shows that, even to the twentieth day of a fast and sometimes thereafter, great amounts of bile and mucus appear in the discharges. The necessity is thus apparent of the daily use of the enema. Repetition insuring thorough cleansing of the colon is most essential in employing the internal bath, for the injection of only a small quantity of water acts detrimentally since it serves to render the contents of the bowel easily absorptive, and is not in amount sufficient to be evacuated freely. For this reason also small enemas occasion weakness in the patient, an additional objection advanced against the use of the injection. Less than three quarts should never be administered at any one time. It may be added that in weakened cases the effort of ejecting the water and the contents of the bowel may be lessened by the insertion of a colon-tube to a depth of approximately six inches into the rectum; through this tube the fluid waste and small particles of fecal matter can pass without difficulty. Hence no matter how weak or depressed the patient may be, the enema is possible of administration with- out undue physical depletion, while the utmost relief always follows the removal of body filth.

Erroneous teaching is responsible for the assertion that the continual use of the enema during a fast or in health will occasion weakness in a patient and lack of function of the colon, and that natural movements of the bowels will not again occur. In other words, that the patient will thereafter be compelled to resort perforce to the internal bath for bowel evacuation. Natural movements of the bowels, as has been said, are directly dependent upon normal digestion, and in a system organically perfect and naturally correct in digestive and assimilative processes, peristalsis and subsequent evacuation of refuse products occur in sequence. No instance of loss of function or of paralysis of the bowel as the result of the judicious use of the internal bath has ever been observed or known in the course of the long experience of the writer. On the contrary, the enema has been found to restore natural action and to act as a tonic stimulus upon the muscles of the colon, preventing all chance of septic poisoning and of resulting disease.

Years of feeding upon other than natural foods and of excess consumption have brought about conditions in the body of man that leave no doubt as to food rubbish retained in the intestinal canal. Its removal is absolutely essential to health, and pure water is the natural agent for the accomplishment of this purpose. When digestive power reasserts itself, the daily use of the enema may be discontinued, but it should without question be administered at least twice weekly in health.

The factors that conduce to decomposition in the colon are several in number. The organ is developed as a storage reservoir for evacuations; it forms a suitable culture medium well supplied with warmth and moisture; and there are microbes constantly present, capable of utilizing toxic substances, and in their turn producing them. Delay in evacuation gives a time of retention sufficient for further microbic propagation. These conditions exist in the normal colon, and, when frequent action is impeded, as in constipation, they increase to the highest degree of development.

A modern scientist, not a physician, Elie Metchnikoff, recently called attention to the fact that extreme longevity in mankind is directly dependent upon the frequency and copiousness of bowel discharges. This view, taken without qualification, may be regarded as extravagant, but there is good reason for accepting his contention that the primary cause of shortness of life is the pernicious action of poisons absorbed from the colon.

Following the medical plan of annihilating the symptom, Metchnikoff sought and supposedly found that constant use of sour milk placed a limit on intestinal fermentation. The active principle in this fluid is an organism known as the bacillus of lactic acid, which Metchnikoff discovered to be antagonistic to the microbes habitually present in the large intestine. He dubbed his fighting ally a "friendly germ." Again the reverse reasoning of medicine is apparent. Why not take steps for the prompt removal of the soil in which "unfriendly germs" propagate, instead of making the colon a battle-ground of which the decomposing dead are a source of further septic poisoning? The enema solves this problem, and a clean bowel, whether it determine long life in itself or not, at least conduces to health and to length of days.

Since the colon and its attachment, the vermiform appendix, are frequently subject to disease, and since the colon itself is the principal source of toxic infection, surgical fanatics argue that these are unnecessary organs, and suggest complete removal. Operations have been performed in which the ileum has been attached directly to the sigmoid flexure, and the entire lower bowel between these points has been extirpated. Surely this is one way of eradicating bowel trouble, since the organ vanishes, but it may be added that the mortality from surgical shock in this triumph of science is ninety-nine percent. The enema will long hold its own in comparison with methods as drastic as this.

CHAPTER IX: FOOD AND DISEASE

'When thou sittest to eat with a ruler, consider diligently what is before thee: And put a knife to thy throat, if thou be a man given to appetite.'

Proverbs XXIII: 1-2

In the life of man tradition, inheritance, and education often combine to foster and preserve doctrines that are misleading. And in no manner is this so well illustrated as in the orthodox methods employed for the relief of bodily ills. By the popular mind disease is contemplated with dread, and, when certain symptoms are in evidence, it is fled from in panic and in terror. This attitude is to be expected so long as present conditions prevail, but the prophecy is ventured that the day is at hand when human ailments will be regarded, as in truth they are, but rational, natural processes of cure. To the general awakening in respect to the preservation of public and individual health, apparent within the past two decades, is due this reasonable view of a most important question.

Disease is not a foe to life, but is the plan of nature instituted to restore a system temporarily unbalanced to equilibrium or health. That the general conception and treatment of disease are wrong, and that health lies within reach of all diseased bodies that are not organically imperfect are truths which, it is hoped, the text will fully demonstrate.

A healthy human organism is one in position to liberate energy and vitality as these forces are needed in the acts that constitute life. To preserve the body in health, man breathes, sleeps, and eats. These are natural laws, and, if any one of them is violated, functional disturbances occur that must result in disease.

Centuries of catering to the sensory organs lie behind modern carelessness in feeding the human body, and custom has caused false standards to be erected about the appetite of man. Food in its preparation has long been subordinated to the sense of taste, and, ingested in excess of the amount required to make good the losses incurred through physical and mental activity, has entailed much un- necessary labor upon the processes of digestion and disposal of waste. Because of almost universal violation of the natural law of nutrition in respect to overeating, this vice, apparent though it be, and weakening and distressing in its effects as it is, calls for correction as does no other in the long list of offenses against nature. From time to time many earnest seekers have advanced beliefs and theories tending to develop a panacea for disease, but so far without success. That relief is to be found is not only probable but certain, since nature deals but in cause and effect, and the tendency in all life is towards perfect bodily balance, without which health is not. One thing, however, is clearly shown in the results of the investigations thus far conducted: The human race possesses the possibility of reaching a point where nutrition and elimination shall become functions automatically performed.

The action of food within the body embodies a process more or less mechanical. Its function consists in replacing cell structure the usefulness of which is exhausted, a function that supplies and repairs the working parts of the human machine. In this process energy is liberated, utilized, and dissipated, and, in so far as the expenditure of what may be called nervous force is compensated, a balance is maintained. To accomplish its work, food must be prepared for conversion into living tissue, and the details of this change are sufficiently familiar to preclude description here. However, the act of digestion is an effort at once nervous and muscular, which will be followed by troubles innumerable if continued beyond the real need of the system; for, when the body is overloaded with sustenance, energy that might well be utilized for other important purposes is employed in the disposal of that in excess of what is needed for the repair of used tissue. Surplus is thus accumulated in circulation, in tissue, and in the organs of elimination; and of this the portion which the liver is able to separate and cast out, together with undigested matter in the intestinal tract, decomposes and is absorbed to be re-deposited with detrimental effect. The natural avenues of energic force are, as a consequence, clogged, imperfect functioning occurs, and disease results.

Normally only that portion of digested food that is assimilated can be used by the blood for the repair of cell structure; the remainder is refuse, and, in cases of overfeeding, it takes its place, as described, with undigested material to ferment and decompose in the intestinal tract. Absorption of toxins thus formed occurs rapidly and continuously, as is shown by the symptoms that follow.

An examination of human fecal discharges in the average case reveals conditions that are conclusive. Undigested food is found, digested food products and old feces are present, and, dependent upon diet and mastication, the odor is more or less offensive. Normal refuse from properly masticated and chemically changed food is not disagreeable in odor. When daily examination is continued for a time, assurance is gained that food is not all digested; that the bowels are not completely cleared of waste by a regular daily movement; that fermenting, rotting matter defiles the human interior to an extent scarcely to be accepted as a fact; and that, in consequence of over-supply, unnecessary tax is put upon the digestive tract and upon the organs of elimination. The results are apparent in a waste of energy that lowers vitality and diminishes the power of assimilation a double injury.

A movement of the bowels each day is no proof of a clean and healthy alimentary canal. Sufferers from digestive troubles often assume that, because the bowels are regular in action, the evacuations are complete and sufficient, forgetful of the fact that, in most instances, but the rectum alone is relieved of its contents. Additional evidence of a filthy internal condition is furnished upon the administration of the enema, when quantities of old, hardened fecal matter appear. And post mortem dissection of the colon gives further proof of foulness, for masses of waste are discovered clinging to its walls, material beyond the power of the organ to eliminate, the direct result of overfeeding. A movement of the bowels in these circumstances takes place only through the center of the clogged tube. These facts are developed in the majority of cases, and but one inference can be made food waste rotting in human intestines forms soil analogous to that of filth decomposing in outer air, with the result that the destroying agents of nature, bacilli, are at once introduced fully equipped as scavengers.

The germ evolves and propagates, not to create disease, but to remove its cause; not on account of the ill-health of the body, but for the sole reason that ignorant and improper handling of the resources of nature furnishes conditions that stimulate and conserve germ life. The remedy lies, not in making the body a battle-ground for myriad antagonistic hordes of minute organisms, but in expeditiously removing the putrid field in which alone these really invaluable servants of nature can exist.

Despite prevalent belief, disease never strikes suddenly, but is the consequence of long-continued violations of natural law. It is the result of a gradual clogging of the avenues of vitality with dead material, a long-drawn process of stifling the forces of life.

"Every disease," says Dr. E. H. Dewey, "is an inherited possibility, which every violation of the laws of life tends to develop. It is never simply an attack on a well person, but rather a summing-up of the more or less life-long violations of health laws." As a result of these transgressions, loss of digestive power occurs; disease symptoms become apparent on lines of least resistance; and the physical scales no longer balance. The decomposition of every morsel of food that enters a human stomach in excess of the need for repair of broken-down tissue and growth is always the direct cause of morbid conditions. Defining disease as here outlined, it may be succinctly stated that it is the result of the products of the decomposition of surplus food held within the body food beyond the need of the system for the repair of broken-down tissue.

Symptoms of disease, the outward and inward evidences of its presence, vary with temperament, hereditary tendencies, surroundings, and the physical condition of the individual. No two human beings ever express identical morbid signs, even in like environment; and the reason underlying the development of disease symptoms, perhaps diametrically opposed, in persons similarly situated, is to be sought in the domain of the phenomena of heredity.

Food prepared in the successive stages of digestion for conversion into tissue nourishment is eventually transformed into chyle, a milky fluid that is absorbed from the intestines and carried through liver, heart, and lungs to the arterial system. Elements other than food products enter into the cell structure, but the great supply of material for rebuilding is secured from food ingested and digested, and blood quality depends in large degree upon food properly converted and perfectly assimilated. Any disturbance of any part of the processes of digestion and assimilation causes an imperfect supply of blood and hence of tissue nourishment. When such disorder occurs, abnormal functioning of vital organs results, the blood becomes encumbered with impurities, and nature at once makes effort to restore normal balance by manifesting disease.

A review of the physiology of the passage of the blood through the body evidences that health is synonymous with perfect blood quality and circulation. What is deposited in one state is removed in another; and, given a pure blood supply properly delivered, broken-down tissue is at once eliminated and replaced. The products of converted food are furnished to the tissue by the blood, and this fluid gathers and carries away the refuse. Upon the normal performance of this process depends the maintenance of the animal body.

With these premises it should not now require an exhaustive argument to establish the fact that disease has its origin in digestion abused and impaired. The treatment herein described rests in its entirety upon the exposition of this fundamental truth, and long experience at various cases places an axiomatic value upon the statement that, whatever the symptom, the sole cause of disease is found in impaired digestion, manifested in impure blood. The law of compensation in nature is here amply and completely shown, for each and every violation of the rule of obedience is visited with condign correction, individual or cumulative. On the other hand, relief and restoration are offered when the road of indulgence is forsaken and natural paths resumed.

Granting that impaired digestion is the source of impure blood or disease, it is the purpose of the following pages to establish that abused digestive functions, relieved from their labors for a time, will recover and return with renewed vigor to their appointed tasks. Rest and rest alone is the one means of recuperation in the realm of nature, and the sole purpose of physical life is so to maintain the structure of the human body that disease may be prevented and eradicated.

CHAPTER X: REST AND ELIMINATION

'A man cannot be a perfect physician of any one save of himself alone.'

Louis Cornaro

Body tissue is continuously undergoing change of structure. The cells that form it are constantly dying, are cast off, and fresh material is supplied. The waste eliminated is poison; and, without muscular rest, this dead and harmful refuse cannot be replaced with sufficient rapidity by new products. This applies not only to muscles in active use, but to all of the bodily fabric. Rapid exercise of any part of the human machine can be continued but for a short time, for, because of vigorous muscular action, voluntary or involuntary, poisonous substances are thrown into the blood and are carried to tissue, nerves, and brain. Through the nerve cells the heart is affected, and the muscles of respiration are to a similar extent disturbed, and resulting symptoms of self-toxication appear that may end in death. The only means of restoration lies in absolute muscular rest.

The heart, though making contractions at the rate of seventy-two beats a minute, is able to continue its work throughout the life of an individual, since each contraction of this muscle is followed by an interval of rest, during which the cells recuperate. Stimulate the heart beats beyond the normal rate, and a point is soon reached at which poisonous products are not replaced by fresh cells, since the intervals of rest are insufficient. Similar conditions are met in the action of the diaphragm and of the chest and abdominal muscles used in respiration.

Just here a distinction in function needs notation:

The muscles that move involuntarily, those that are not subject to the human will, never know absolute rest, for they continue their labors whether the body be asleep or awake.

On the other hand, those muscles, the action of which depends upon the direction of the human will, cannot work continuously, lest fatigue with fatal exhaustion follow.

Seemingly, automatic labor, labor not directed by the highest function of consciousness, does not wear. It is only conscious work that requires for recuperation and muscle-rebuilding other means than simple non-use or physical rest. This is granted in that loss of consciousness, regularly recurrent in animal life, which is called sleep.

All during life each component part of the body in the very act of living produces poison within itself. When toxins accumulate faster than they are eliminated, as occurs when no interval of rest is granted, fatigue is felt, and fatigue is only another name for toxic infection. A normal amount of labor is easily cared for by the muscular system, but excess work brings disaster.

If action and rest are so regulated that the cells may give off their waste products at a rate to keep pace with new formations, muscle, and nerve tissue as well, will always be in position to liberate energy on demand.

From the time of birth until death, the organs of the human body function continuously. On the other hand, in the vegetable kingdom the plant maintains and conserves life by added growth from year to year. The vital parts of the plant are re-created and their predecessors become mere physical supports corresponding to the bony framework in man. The power resident in the tree of producing new equipment annually is denied to humanity, not by nature, but because of imperfect interpretation of natural law. Physical growth and muscular development in man are never completely rounded out, and this may be attributed to a double cause. Theoretically, every muscle of the body should be exercised impartially and be nourished with just the quantity of cell pabulum that is necessary for the replacement of its waste. This never occurs; but it is a possibility that may be contemplated with surety since it is a natural condition. To bring it to pass, reciprocal action must exist between intake and outgo, rebuilding and waste, labor and rest, consciousness and sleep.

The processes of nutrition are involuntary in character so long as material is supplied for their use, but they may be directed by the individual to the extent of the selection and preparation of nourishment. In this they differ from the functions of the involuntary muscles and organs of the body, the control of which is entirely beyond that of the human will. When through abuse the digestive function becomes impaired, disease results. Functional disease is then analogous to muscular fatigue, and, since nature knows but one law of recuperation that of rest it is reasonable to assume what the text promulgates: Rest through abeyance of the processes of digestion offers the possibility of complete renewal of functional machinery.

The manner in which the digestive organs may be given needed rest is perhaps not at once apparent. The mere thought of abstention from food carries with it violation of long-taught doctrine that frequent feeding in sickness and in health is necessary for the maintenance of vitality and strength. Yet just this omission of food is meant when rest through abeyance of the digestive function is suggested. The phenomena of fasting for the cure of disease include facts that prove that the human body does not depend for strength or for vitality upon ingested food; the latter is utilized for the repair of the body as the vehicle of the expression of these forces, and by it the material framework is kept in condition to liberate the life principle in its variety of manifestation.

In illness weight is always lost, and, contingent upon the duration or the severity of disease, the substance of the body diminishes in greater or in less degree. During sickness, under prevailing methods, feeding is continuous, and, if the stomach rebel, nutrient enemata are pressed into service.

The question suggests itself, why, if food is constantly supplied, naturally or otherwise, does the body lose in weight? The answer is found in the fact that the intake is not digested, consequently is not assimilated, and, far from nourishing the tissues, is an added burden to functions already overtaxed. An- other cause is discovered in that brain and nerve tissue, as instruments for the expression of thought and sensation, are protected from deterioration in substance, even in disease, by a provision of nature that permits them to utilize nourishment stored in the interstices of body tissue. This they consume in illness and in health, and, when in disease a normal balance is not preserved, when cells are not rebuilt as waste occurs, they still are supported from this source.

With slight differences the physiology of digestion in all mammals is markedly similar. When disease is manifest, the lower animals and the reptiles abstain from food until health is restored. They are compelled to this by instinct, a force implanted by nature in the whole of animate creation. The fasting which animals instinctively undergo is a fact that is constantly observed, but not in general intelligently perceived. A common expression of the stable in reference to the ailments of the horse embodies the phrase, "off his feed," and this alone illustrates the instinct that impels the animal to fast when its physical well-being is disturbed. A python in captivity has been known to abstain from food for thirteen months with no deleterious effects beyond a loss in weight; and cats often prolong abstention to skeleton condition, when they rapidly return to health with strength and vigor increased. Instances such as these may be multiplied indefinitely.

Omitting the mental states of fear and worry, which of necessity react upon the physical body, and bodily conditions of severe pain or of continued exposure, the average human being cannot die from want of food for several months. This fact has been substantiated in many instances in medical history, and it is verified and corroborated daily in fasting for the cure of disease.

If, then, the body can exist without food for a time, and, if in illness the stomach instinctively objects to its introduction, it is reasonable to infer that food not desired is not necessary, and, once accepted, this inference is abundantly justified. The results of its practical application are such that they lead to the conclusion that, in the absence of mechanical defects in physical organs, abstinence from food, with other natural health-giving and health-preserving accompaniments, is the unfailing remedy for the cure of functional ills.

CHAPTER XI: AUXILIARIES IN FASTING

'The heart receiveth benefit or harm most from the air which we breathe.
'Washing the body in water is good for length of life.
'Sleep doth supply somewhat to nourishment, and conferreth to length of days.
'No body can be healthy without exercise, neither natural body nor politic.'

Lord Bacon

Breathing. Nature has provided in the air that surrounds the earth a plentiful supply of oxygen, a gas that is essential to the maintenance of human life. Its function lies in replacing carbonic acid, a poisonous gas developed within the body by the breaking down of tissue, and delivered to the lungs in venous blood. In the process of breathing, oxygen is inhaled and appropriated, while carbonic acid is expelled. The act of respiration exposes the blood to the air, and by mutual diffusion the two operations of oxygenating the blood and freeing it from carbonic acid are accomplished at one and the same time. The muscular movements of respiration are not dependent upon the will, as the same process goes on in sleep and in other unconscious states. The number of respiratory movements in health varies from fourteen to eighteen per minute, and besides carbonic acid, watery vapor and a small quantity of organic matter are exhaled, the latter dependent upon the condition of the digestive apparatus.

In order to supply oxygen to the system, from 300 to 400 cubic feet of air are drawn into the lungs in twenty-four hours. Each hour an adult inhales about 500 grains of oxygen and emits about 600 grains of carbonic acid with a much larger amount of watery vapor. Deprived of air the body perishes from asphyxiation.

It follows that not only is a continued supply of fresh air essential to life, but that constant care is necessary to insure its purity at the moment of delivery. The natural channels for the passage of air to the lungs begin at the nostrils, which are furnished with short fine hairs and with mucus secretion, mechanical preventives of the inhalation of dust and light material. If obstruction of the nasal tract occurs, it is possible for breathing to take place through the mouth, but so harmful is the latter method to general health that attention is here directed to its results.

Overfeeding a child invariably develops a cold with accompanying nasal discharge and consequent obstruction of the natural air passages. A prolonged cold or a series of colds compel the use of the mouth for the act of breathing, a method that, if not corrected, eventually becomes habitual. Constant irritation and inflammation of the mucus membrane of the nostrils and of the vault of the pharynx cause the much discussed adenoid growths to form, and obstruction of the air canal is thereafter permanent until removal of the obstacles is accomplished either by the fast or by surgical means. Children thus affected are stupid and sluggish and exhibit a characteristic facial expression approaching that of imbecility. In fact, when the habit of mouth breathing has been contracted in infancy or in adult life, even when no obstruction of the nasopharyngeal vault exists, not only do the nasal passages, through the lack of exercise, fail of normal development, but the open mouth and dulled eyes denote a serious deficiency in intellectual advance and capability.

We cannot know the exact source whence is received the influx of vitality and energy, the expression of which is life, nor in what manner these forces penetrate the physical body and animate its movements and its thought, but whatever is gained of vital power from without and life is very evidently neither residual nor developed within the body must reach us from the domain of the surrounding atmosphere, either through air itself or through its penetrating medium, ether. Its transference to the brain directly through the bony structure immediately above and back of the nasal passages is conceivable; and, while the purity of the atmospheric constituents that furnish the lungs with blood-restoring activity may well be vitiated in transmission by paths not naturally intended, the lack of intellectuality displayed in all mouth breathers cannot be accounted for on this basis, since no depreciation in blood value is apparent. Hence the theory here presented: that vital force enters the body from without, through the natural air passages and the bony cavities immediately above and in their rear. Whatever the attitude of the reader in respect to this, there can be no question of the importance to be attached to the formation of a nasal breathing habit hygienic, because it is natural; healthful, because it is correct.

In the fast proper respiratory methods must be pursued, and deep breathing practiced. Every portion of the lung surface should be exposed to the general purification resultant from oxygenation of the blood, and an insure this, in addition to lung exercise, the body should be in contact with outer air day and night. Well ventilated living and sleeping rooms are important to the highest degree in illness, in fasting, and in health.

Bathing. The skin or covering of the human body consists of an outer layer called the cuticle, and of an inner one, the corium. These constitute the true skin, but under them lies a third layer of cellular tissue, which is considered also as part of the skin, when that word is used in its most comprehensive sense. In man the skin is covered more or less with scattered hairs, profuse in some parts and scanty in others. The office of the skin is one of protection to the organs beneath, and it is also a vast excretory system, sending out quantities of perspiration through the sudoriferous glands located in its texture. Each of these glands consists of a long fine tube coiled into a knot near its closed end, which is situated in the cutaneous cellular tissue, and constitutes the gland proper, and of a straight or spinal duct traversing the outer layers and ending in a surface opening called a pore. Nearly 3,000 of the latter are found upon a square inch of the palm of the hand, and at least 500 on an equal space upon other parts of the body.

Perspiration is the watery matter "breathed out" from the system through the pores described. It is more copious than the exudation from the lungs by respiration, but the quantity discharged varies greatly, and is affected by the heat or the dryness of the atmosphere, by liquids drunk, by exercise, and by the relative activity of the kidneys. Sensible perspiration is that which is perceptible in the form of small drops, but by far the larger portion exuded is of the insensible or non-visible kind. Solid matter is carried to the surface of the skin in the sweat, and authorities all agree that a considerable proportion of the total waste of the body is evacuated in this manner. Hence, besides keeping the skin in a healthy, moist condition, and acting through evaporation as a refrigerator regulating body temperature, perspiration takes its share in the elimination of useless material.

Close sympathy exists between the skin and the lungs, the kidneys, the liver, and the bowels, and this is evidenced in the fact that, when one or other of these organs becomes affected by disease, the perspiratory function is sympathetically deranged and vice versa. This does not necessarily mean that the effect is produced by physical transference of suppressed exhalation to the internal organ nor the reverse; the chief impression seems to be made upon the nervous system. But the importance of the relation existing between the skin and the other excretory organs is such that it cannot be disregarded when disease is to be remedied.

In order to insure functional activity of the surface of the body, frequent bathing is necessary at all times. For this purpose one cleansing bath daily is required. Dead, scaly particles of skin, dirt, and the products of perspiration are thus removed, and the other organs of elimination are relieved from the performance of extra labor. The rule of the body is that of cleanliness, internal and external. The importance of the daily cleansing bath during a fast period needs no further exposition.

A bath with temperature ranging from 80 to 90 degrees Fahrenheit is suitable for elderly people and for those who do not nervously react with promptness from either heat or cold. One of temperature not more than 105 degrees is cleansing in the highest sense if soap be freely used and the flesh-brush vigorously plied. The cold bath of register lower than 75 degrees should never be employed except in health and for tonic purposes. It has a powerful stimulating action on the circulation and nervous system, in addition to but slight cleansing properties. It cannot be used during the fast.

Bathing should never be undertaken immediately before or directly after eating, and an interval of at least two hours should elapse between. During the menstrual flow in woman, medical authority to the contrary, a warm sitz or full body bath, with a warm vaginal douche are imperative for cleanliness and for relief and ease in function.

Caution is directed in connection with all bathing toward continuing the bath to undue length. Only time sufficient to cleanse the body or to receive a tonic effect should be occupied; more than this is weakening. When, in the fast, chilliness occurs, a few minutes in the hot bath equalizes the circulation and remedies the condition, care being taken to guard against exposure at its conclusion.

Civilization and the customs it entails are responsible for many physiological evils. The two great mediums through which energy is delivered to the human body, pure air and sunshine, are in large part denied immediate contact with its surface. Clothing prevents full elimination of perspiration and its products, which remain to be partially absorbed or to clog the pores of the skin. This defect can be remedied to a degree by daily exposing the naked body to the outer air for as long a time as can be spared from other duties. The air bath is a valuable adjunct to natural treatment for the prevention and cure of disease, and of equal worth is the action of the direct rays of the sun upon the skin. The human plant absorbs the tonic properties of air and sunlight with the eagerness of its garden counterpart, and these baths add their quota of benefits to the other hygienic means described. In the fast these two baths should form a daily habit.

The skin is the natural clothing of the body. Its protection to the parts beneath is aided by deposits of fat, a non-conductor of heat, distributed more or less uniformly over the body. When overheated, evaporation of perspiration cools; when chilled, closed pores retain the body warmth. Like the lungs, the skin admits of blood oxygenation through the walls of the capillaries, and, as has been shown, it is an organ of elimination as well.

In the conservation of body heat, the skin is the thermostat of the organism. It preserves and regulates temperature, and acts as a governor of internal mechanism. If its function be interfered with by the interposition of substances between it and outer air, evaporation cannot take place freely, and elimination of the products of the pores is impeded, if not entirely arrested. Temperature is maintained in this instance artificially and abnormally, for disease of function causes interior combustion that is detrimental to health. Kindred organs are called upon to do the work of body covering, and danger lurks in forced exertion. A chill precedes a fever; the pores are closed; intense heat is generated; the fever is cured when perspiration with subsequent evaporation is restored. A very striking exemplification of these facts is given in cases of cutaneous burns where large areas are affected. Respiration is in- creased to exhaustion, and kidney discharges are highly colored with waste that ordinarily is eliminated through the pores. If an extreme proportion of skin area is seared, suffocation ensues. Also fatal results ensue when the body is covered with a substance that is impervious to air, such as gold-leaf. Here the symptoms are those that accompany asphyxiation.

Ages of submission to conventionality have compelled skin covering, and have evolutionally made of this organ a partial functioner. Since clothing is an essential of civilization, the remedy lies in making it as light and as pervious to air as is consistent with decency, and in caring for the surface of the body with constancy and diligence.

Sleep. Nature's law of recuperation is that of rest, of relief from labor. The instrument of thought and of motive government, the brain, obtains its repose in regularly recurring periods of unconsciousness and cessation of bodily activity the hours of sleep. It is then that the cells of the human battery are recharged, that the working principal receives its potential for transformation during conscious moments. Sleep is a physiological necessity and death results within a few days if it be denied. In the fast, due to slight brain congestion produced by excessive elimination in the prior stages, inability to slumber is sometimes present, but attention to the bath and to the ventilation of the sleeping apartment brings refreshing rest as disease departs. No garment worn during the day should cover the body in sleep, and bed clothing should be regulated to an accurate degree of protection, neither too heavy nor too light.

Exercise. The maintenance of every muscle and organ of the body in proportionate development is regulated by its work. Constant use of a particular muscle adds to its substance at the expense of that of its neighbor, hence the aim of all exercise should be directed at equality of labor. Trunk and legs, arms and neck, all should receive proportioned attention. Muscular development also depends upon an unimpeded circulation of blood and upon healthful cell-forming constituents constantly furnished to replace used tissue. Constriction of the body in any part prevents free circulation, and only loose garments permit of full growth and proper development. The tight collar, the garter, and the corset, make flabby muscles inevitable, and only a body unrestrained by the bonds of conventional dress can hope for physical perfection in form. But few elderly women of the present day can exhibit an abdomen that is not pendulous, nor breasts that do not sag; and, as age creeps on, thighs and buttocks droop with muscular atrophy and with deposits of adipose cells. The possibilities of natural hygienic living, coupled with judicious exercise, are surely worth consideration, if merely for the satisfaction of personal appearance, but their more important effects upon general health and longevity make neglect of these desiderata sinful and criminal.

During a fast moderate exercise in keeping with the daily access of strength is advised, and after its completion constant comprehensive muscular activity is essential to rebuilding and to form-development.

The subject matter of this chapter, then, resolves itself into three requisites, equally divided in importance:

Ventilation of the body within and without; Activity for its members; and Rest for their recuperation.

Of similar moment are these hygienic measures with the laws of maintenance elsewhere enumerated.

CHAPTER XII: DIET

*'Know prudent, cautious self-control
   Is wisdom's root.'*

Robert Burns

Diet at any time is largely a matter of special need, but it would seem that, after a course of fasting, the successful issue of which depends upon a reduction to normal in all respects, certain fixed rules might be laid down to apply to all cases. Peculiar limitations are developed in each individual, for which the physical sins of generations of ancestors are in great measure responsible; hence empirical methods must be employed in the selection of foods requisite for the case in hand.

Taste plays an important part in the choice of food material in health, and it is popularly believed that, when an article of sustenance is not repugnant to this sense, it is healthful and wholesome, and that harm cannot result from its ingestion. One of the objects that nature has in placing the nerves of taste in the mouth is to prevent noxious substances from entering the stomach; but, as a consequence of persistent cultivation, the sense of taste has been much perverted, and most men and women are more or less abnormal in taste perception. To the lack of sense perception in this respect is due much of carelessness in mastication. Improperly accomplished salivation and the seeds of disease are resulting evils. With normal taste the medical profession would be at loss to administer the average drug were the patient to masticate or insalivate its substance. Recognizing this fact as well as the subsequent action of the digestive juices upon medical remedies, the physician obviates the difficulty presented by the use of capsules or by introducing the drug directly into the blood.

The sense of smell, reaching out beyond the body ere food material passes the lips, assists in its selection, and it and taste, when normal in function and not vitiated by cultivation and habit, form a perfect picket-line of protection against the introduction of unwholesome nourishment into the system. Normally constituted bodies prefer those odors that are classified as pleasant, yet continual personal contact with emanations that are distinctly disagreeable, first brings tolerance and finally pleasure in their presence.

Perhaps this departure from natural law and normal instinct can be illustrated in convincing form by contemplating the sensual delight of the epicure in cheeses of doubtful age but of indubitable rottenness.

The fallacy of attempting practical application of a theory of food selection based upon taste and smell alone is easily demonstrated. The question resolves itself into one concerning the needs of the body, but, after a fast, taste and smell are restored to normal acuteness and, so long as they remain in this state, they may be used as partial indicators. At this time all wholesome food gives delight and is desired with a hunger created in a clean, healthy system that asks for nourishment and that fully enjoys its ingestion. Simple foods, properly prepared and correctly proportioned as to the relative amounts of fats, carbo-hydrates, and protein, with the necessary mineral salts, are what the dietitian and the patient should endeavor to supply. The fast is ended, the system cleansed, and the digestive organs are in full vigor, waiting to form pure blood and pure tissue from pure food.

No further detail is needed to show that mankind habitually overeats and that, as a result, nutritive material is absorbed into the circulation in quantity beyond the requirements of the body, loading the system with an unnecessary and harmful burden and hampering with poisonous waste the operation of its machinery. But, just as the liver stands guard, in so far as it may, over matters absorbed, and just as it separates the good from the bad, so, at the very inception of the digestive process, the mouth, with its armor of teeth and its salivary apparatus, determines in large degree the amount of food needed in nutrition.

The mouth holds the nerves of taste, taste is enjoyed in the mouth, and taste has its great purpose in deciding just when food has been ground between the teeth sufficiently to prepare it for the subsequent processes. Taste disappears when food has been properly insalivated, and too thorough mastication cannot occur, for the benefits derived are immeasurable, even apart from the comminution of solids. The mouth easily accomplishes this work when the habit of mastication has been acquired, but, if it perform it carelessly, the other organs of digestion cannot act in normal function, and, as a matter of fact, perfect digestion cannot occur, since one of its processes has been omitted. The only portion of the operation of digestion that can be voluntarily controlled is that which is done in the mouth, hence the subject of the mastication of food is an all-important one. Its value in the economy of the human body is excellently treated by Horace Fletcher in his "*A-B-Z of our own Nutrition*."

Fletcher says: "When food is filtered into the body after having become liquefied and made alkaline or at least neutral by saliva, the appetite is given a chance to measure the needs of the body and to discriminate against excess. As soon as the point of complete saturation of any one deficiency is reached, the appetite is cut off as short as possible, with no indication of stomach fullness. It will welcome a little of protein, and then turn to sugar or fat in some of their numerous forms. Thirst for water will assert itself for a moment, sometimes asking but a drop and again for a full glass; and, afterwards, when near the point of complete saturation, appetite will hesitate for a moment, as if searching around for some rare substance and may find its final satisfaction in a single spoonful of sweet, or of a sip of something in sight.

"The appetite, satisfied by the infiltering process, is a sweetly appeased appetite, calm, rested, contented, normal. There is no danger from the flooding of intemperance for there is not even toleration of excess, either of more food or of more drink, and this contented appetite will remain in the condition of contentment until another need has really been earned by evaporation or destructive katabolism."

Fletcher uses in his description the term, appetite, in the sense that the word, hunger, is employed in the present text. In the conditions that he so well expresses lies the solution of the problem of overeating. Mastication, carried to the degree that taste is neutralized, absolutely precludes eating save for the needs of metabolism. The supply is made equal to the demand, neither more nor less; and intemperance in food or drink is effectively prevented.

A scientific discussion of the question of diet is manifestly out of place in this text. Authorities differ widely and none has dealt with feeding from the viewpoint met after a fast, with a stomach, so to speak, re-created.

It is no undue iteration to again point out that diet is largely a matter of special need, and that no fixed rules can be promulgated to apply in every case; but certain general principles require discussion, of which the first and most important deals with the use or non-use of meat. Flesh in any form should never enter the dietary of normal man. Arguments for and against have long been exchanged on this subject, and advocates of the strongest will combat the non-flesh diet for years to come. The argument that serves to refute this error in hygiene contains, among others, the following premises: First, dead animal tissue holds within it the products of metabolism. The process of change is suddenly arrested when the animal is killed, and the juices of the body of the latter contain un-eliminated toxic products from broken-down cell-tissue that no process of cooking can destroy. For that matter, even were they completely annihilated, flesh is still changed vegetable tissue with the waste of the process of change and that of the living organism retained in its structure, a condition that logically suggests the consumption of the plant rather than of its creation. In addition, decomposition of animal flesh begins at the moment of death, and by the time it is consumed as food, decay has progressed almost to the point of putrefaction. In the fast it is observed that excessive meat eaters and patients who previously have undergone the "Salisbury treatment" with its forced feeding of flesh, exhibit a foulness in elimination so much beyond that in all other cases that it renders them obnoxious even to themselves.

Mr. Otto Carque in his "Errors of Bio-Chemistry" says: "There is also a marked physiological difference between plant and animal food. Animals are distinguished from vegetables by incessant decay in every tissue, a decay which is proportional to animal activity. This incessant decay necessitates incessant repair, so that the animal body has been likened to a temple on which two opposite forces are at work in every part, the one tearing down, the other repairing the breach as fast as it is made. In plants no such incessant decay has ever been discovered. If it exists at all, it must be very trifling in comparison. Protoplasm, it is true, is taken from the older parts of the plant, and these parts die; but the protoplasm does not seem to decompose, but is used again for tissue building. Thus the eternal activity of animals is of two kinds, tissue-destroying and tissue-building, while that of plants is principally of one kind, tissue building. Flesh foods will, therefore, impart less vitality to our system than plant foods, because the former always contain a quantity of substances which have undergone the various stages of katabolism and have lost their vital force.

We feel drowsy and indolent after a heavy meal of meat, while an apple, an orange, a bunch of grapes, instantly refreshes us. The theories that flesh makes flesh, that blood is converted into blood, that calf's or sheep's brain increases our mental capacity, that meat is predigested plant food, cannot stand in the light of physiological chemistry."

And again, recent experiments carried out most thoroughly by Irving Fisher, Professor of Political Economy at Yale University, show beyond any chance of refutation that the physical endurance of the human body is increased to the utmost by non-flesh diet. In the course of these experiments meat-eating athletes competed in test exercises with non-meat eaters, both sedentary and active in occupation. The results were so largely in favor of the non-flesh diet that the most ardent advocates of the opposite side can find no loop-hole through which to escape from the facts.

No adequate explanation is as yet available of the evident superiority of a vegetarian diet over one of flesh as regards endurance, save, perhaps, in the theory that a diet composed in greater part of proteid produces uric acid and other crystalline substances, which in turn cause muscular fatigue in exercise. The facts are patent in these instances as related, as well as in the experiments made by the author of the text along similar lines during the past twelve years. The results obtained demonstrate that a non-flesh diet builds a consistently strong and enduring physical structure, while the reverse is true in great part when meat figures in the list of food ingested. In the past, facts such as these have been obscured and the truth has suffered because the idea contained in the term, "vegetarian," suggested what was popularly regarded as fanaticism carried beyond all bounds. In the history of the world no doctrine advanced with polemical warmth and coupled with enthusiasm and dogma almost religious, has ever had influence upon scientific thought, and, for this reason, the matter needs to be approached deliberately and dispassionately, and with the seriousness befitting a subject that is of more practical import than any other in the whole range of hygienic research. When this shall have been accomplished, the theory embodied in the results of the tests mentioned will be fully borne out and conclusively established as a living truth.

With the individual himself rests the selection of a healthful and properly distributed food supply. In order to maintain a normal body in perfect equilibrium, the amount and the selection of food require careful consideration. Quantity depends upon physical characteristics and the kind of labor at which the subject is employed. A working man destroys more tissue in shorter time than does the banker or the clerk; yet, usually, the latter eat no fewer meals nor less at a sitting than their burly brother. What is needed for the one is far more than sufficient for the others. Should the brain-worker devote spare time to outdoor recreation or to manual labor a mean might be established; but, in general, equilibrium is seldom reached, and the supply of food is far in excess of requirement. The laboring man, too, is at fault in this respect, for, unless his be an exceptional case, the basis of diet is starch, which carries its nutritive principle in a bulky vehicle, demanding extra labor from the digestive tract in order to separate waste from nutriment and to eliminate the former.

To reduce the supply of food to the reciprocal basis of demand, the plan that suggests the omission of the early morning breakfast is perhaps the easiest method to follow, and, once the habit is acquired, this meal is scarcely missed. Common sense indicates that food ingested soon after rising is really detrimental to the body and the mind, for the brain and the nervous system are recuperated by the night's rest, and tissue cells have been replaced while the body slept. In fact, the reasoning power is retarded and hampered in its action by the presence of food in the stomach, since the latter calls energy elsewhere and deprives the brain of just so much of its motive power. The whole mental and nervous systems are at their maximum of energy in the early morning; the blood, in its double function, has replaced the waste it has carried away, and the entire human fabric stands at the threshold of the day ready for anything but the process of digesting food. There is no true hunger at this time; habit alone causes fictitious desire.

Hunger determines the hours for the ingestion of food each day. Regularity of habit as to the times for serving meals is an outgrowth of economic convenience, and more often than not the participant is imposing a burden upon a system in no need, therefore with no desire of sustenance. In health, dependent upon occupation, hunger makes demand at least once but not more than twice daily, if the previous demand has been satisfied.

In much that has been written concerning the matter of diet there are so many sweeping and conflicting statements, impossible rules, and foolish conclusions, that no wonder is felt at the fact that the whole subject is usually ignored as too intricate. There are many who try to enforce personal ideas upon others in this connection; very persistent people these, to whom the term, "crank," may well be applied, and a "crank," who has picked up some scientific jargon and thinks himself cured of his ailments, works more harm than good in the world. This class may be extended to include those who really have been benefited by a diet that happens to suit personal requirements, and it comprises also the one-food people who are in continual search of what not to devour, and who would reduce the universe to whole wheat and pecans. By these, at each encounter with their fellowmen, are discovered disease symptoms identical with their own, for which the same remedy is insisted upon and perhaps applied. It is absurd for any who are not familiar with the chemistry of foods to endeavor to talk learnedly of their action in human economy, and it may be taken as an axiom that, within the individual capacity, which can be known only by individual experiment, a diet limited in variety to not more than three proportioned items at each meal is more conducive to health than unlimited choice or a single dish. A list that is strictly limited to few things trains the stomach to adapt itself accordingly, and eventually trouble ensues when change is attempted.

After all, the amount of food and the kind thereof are of secondary importance to the physical condition of the digestive apparatus of the subject. It must continually be borne in mind that the state of the digestive organs is the crux of the whole situation. Therein lies health or illness. The aim of physician and of patient should constantly be directed at the restoration of the system to health, after which its maintenance in this condition requires careful attention to the selection and to the quantity of food.

CHAPTER XIII: MENTAL AND BODILY REACTION

'Whosoever is out of patience, is out of possession of his body and his soul.'

Lord Bacon

Bodily action may be brought about in two ways through the brain, or through internal or external physical causes. In either case the nerve centers perform their functions, either in the inception of the thought or in the transfer of outward or inward cause. The act of moving the hand may originate in the brain, or it may occur through the fact that the member is in close proximity to fire. In the former circumstance the act begins with the thought in the brain, and nervous influence operates directly upon moving muscles. In the second condition the sensory nerves inform the brain that the flesh is burning, and the brain sets in motion the muscles necessary to move the hand. In both instances the moving power emanates from the brain, and the phenomenon as described may happen in connection with any specific portion of the body. Not only are these facts true of the voluntary muscles, but they may also be observed in similar phase in heart, lungs, stomach, and the organs of function in general. Swallowing an emetic causes vomiting, an effect brought about through muscular convulsion of the stomach for the purpose of ejecting a substance irritating to its nerves. The mere sight or thought of a disgusting object may have the same consequence, and imagination is oftentimes able to produce results like that occasioned by a powerful drug or by a combination of physical conditions.

Every organic act, healthy or diseased, is due solely to a current sent from one of the great nerve centers, and the latter may be called into being either indirectly by reflex action, or directly by feeling or thought. Though the mind and the emotions have large influence over physical functions, the field of operation over which that influence extends is comparatively little known. It is, in some respects, almost unbounded, for every bodily function may be hastened, retarded, or even totally suspended, and life itself may be destroyed by the subjective effect of thought. Pleasurable emotions are physically healthful; painful ones the reverse; but, when too intense and sudden, either can terminate life.

The fibers of the pneumogastric nerve are distributed principally in and about the lungs and the stomach; hence its name. Whatever may be the motor functions that this nerve supplies, it largely influences the progress of digestion, for, when its fibers are cut below those branches that extend to the trachea, digestion is virtually arrested. Nervous influence is essential to the proper action of the stomach, and, in the region of this organ, the nerves are so interlaced one with the other that, even though the direct road be destroyed, by-paths will still remain for the passage of nerve energy. If the latter were not needed in digestion, no reason would exist for the suspension of function by its withdrawal, and the invariable effect of worry, anxiety, fright, and anger is to arrest for a time all digestive action. The cause is obvious when the close connection between the brain and the nerve ganglia is considered. If nervous force is diverted in directions other than those followed in the digestion of food, exactly similar results occur as when the pneumogastric nerve is severed.

Does the physical condition of the body in like manner affect the mind? Observation shows not only that it does influence brain function, but that the results of disease are always and continuously displayed mentally. In many of the ordinary hypochondriacal disturbances, in melancholia, and in the various manias, other forms of treatment should be accompanied by correction of deranged digestive function.

In health the constructive and destructive changes that take place in the human body progress without noticeable diminution or increase in excellence of brain quality, so long as waste material is promptly removed and suitable food is supplied and properly assimilated.

In conditions of debility and weakness, whenever the influx is too large for the demand, or the waste too great for disposal by the organs of elimination, absorption of the poisons generated in fermenting food rubbish retained in the intestinal tract is continuously occurring, and the subject becomes a victim of auto-intoxication, is drunk with the products of his own decomposition. This condition, if long continued, is no less baneful in effect than that of alcoholic saturation, and, in some cases, it may take the form of insanity, while, in all, diminished brain power is evident.

The digestion of a meal, with the subsequent forcing of food waste through the bowels, consumes brain energy in greater amount than does any ordinary work of muscle or of mind, and the result is apparent in weakened vitality, which overfeeding never fails to show. Sufficient food, perfectly digested, produces a body with brain equal to clear thought and maximum of energy. More than this entails excessive labor upon the organs of digestion and consequent overtax of vitality.

The cause of mental disease is one and the same with that of physical disturbance. The physical signs precede the mental danger signals and should be heeded and remedied when first displayed.

The close connection between mental and physical functions is always prominently exhibited in the consequences of the fast, and never more so than in the treatment of those morbid depressions that often lead to confinement in state institutions. These cases originate in the abuse of the digestive organs, which, coupled with hereditary tendencies, affects the nerve centers and ultimately the brain. During the fast constant improvement in mental capacity is shown after proper preparation on restricted diet and omitted meals; and, as the fast progresses, the return to sanity proceeds at a rate commensurate with physical advance. A general fact observed in treating this symptom of disease, when functional in origin, is the presence of quantities of dark, foul-smelling discharges from the bowels, which do not decrease, either in amount or in vileness, until long after the period indicated in ordinary disease. The value of the fast as employed in cases of extreme nervousness and of insanity from functional causes, is almost unknown to alienists, but in the near future it is bound to receive recognition as a certain means of cure.

Due to superficial observation of the delirium of auto-intoxication sometimes present in the early stages of the fast, the criticism has been advanced that prolonged abstinence from food not only produces weakened mentality in the patient, but that it will eventually cause insanity. Fasting never entails a loss of mental power, and this statement is based upon experience gathered from considerably over two thousand cases of fasting in which not one developed aught but improvement in brain function.

All functional derangements, when not corrected, finally lead to organic disease.

In organic disease some portion of the bodily machinery is unable to perform its work; its structure is injured or essentially imperfect.

In functional disease, the structure of the organ shows no defect, yet it is inefficient in action because of nerve force impeded.

It is an established fact that drugs do not affect brain structure; and it is equally well known that, in most instances, insanity causes no deterioration in nerve tissue. In these facts lies strong collateral proof that the sources of mental disease are to be sought elsewhere than in the brain. Injuries and ailments that involve change in brain substance will necessarily interfere with brain function, and, in softening of nerve tissue or in any inflammation, there are organic alterations that may be seen and noted. Incidentally these defects are primarily due to continued functional disease. But in hysteria, epilepsy, and mania, no changes in structure in brain and nerve substance can be discovered, notwithstanding the presence of extreme mental disorder. It may be deduced that a functionally perfect brain is the product of a physically perfect body.

To illustrate the effect of abnormal physical conditions upon mind-function, the following case is cited: The patient, a man thirty years of age, presented himself with a history of continuous digestive trouble, accompanied with strongly developed mental disturbance. Examination created the impression that the disease of the mind was the direct result of functional inactivity of the digestive tract, complicated with decided organic symptoms. A tentative diet of fruit juices and vegetable broths afforded the relief usual when organic labor is progressively decreased. Experience is needful to distinguish between temporary mitigation of the distress of disease and progress towards cure, and, though the symptoms were favorable to the extent of raising the belief in the mind of the patient that recovery would ensue, no definite hope was extended. At the end of four weeks of preparatory treatment, the patient ceased his visits, and a month later his body was found, dead by suicide, an act committed, as its condition showed, within a few days after discontinuing treatment. The actions of the man throughout, together with the contents of a letter found on his person, were evidence that decided lack of mental balance existed, and search of his effects brought to light numbers of long, rambling, scribbled comments that left no doubt concerning mental decay. The body was in shape such that post mortem examination was possible, and the autopsy revealed the following: The kidneys were normal. The lungs and the heart were congested, but functionally equal to their tasks. The liver was cirrhosed, and there was only a rudimentary gall sac, not larger than the first joint of the adult index finger, containing no bile and with no evidence that it had been functioning, since no stain was present, and the color of the sac was a perfect white. The stomach was enlarged to the capacity of four fluid quarts, and it lay in the abdominal cavity opposite the navel; it was filled with food, and all evidences pointed to the fact that glandular function had been inoperative for months. The small intestines were tangled and knotted into a mass, with bleached portions that had been inactive for a long time. The colon was excessively dilated, and its transverse section had fallen, shaping the organ into a letter "M" with the vertex of the dropped tube resting upon the bladder and the pelvic bones; the transverse, ascending, and descending parts adhered at their angles for several inches. The bladder was normal. The pancreas was a soft disintegrated mass. The spleen was extremely large and cirrhosed. The mesentery exhibited old lesions, while no trace of the omentum remained. The brain was structurally perfect.

The above instance of a body exceedingly deformed internally was preserved with its handicaps for thirty years. The cause of the organic defects is to be attributed to digestive functions paralyzed in early life by disease and by the administration of drugs as a remedy. In this case progressive inability to function brought about morbid mental disturbance. It may be asked why this effect was not produced in each of the instances cited under another heading, and reply is made that these also showed the influences of physical condition upon mind-function, but in lesser degree. And the general conclusion is stated that all disease, functional as well as organic, acts detrimentally upon brain capability.

The work that the brain can perform is dependent upon the physical condition of the body. To repeat, a functionally perfect brain is the product of a physically perfect body, but the brain is not a producer of energy, nor of vitality, nor of mental processes. It acts merely as a medium of reception and transmission, and it no more thinks than do the words that express a thought. Mind, as received from the creative source is perfect. Its expression is affected by functional ability or inability in the human instrument.

The mysterious forces, energy and vitality, which are manifested as life, exist outside of and independent of the human body. A healthy organism is one that is in position to liberate these forces in the form of strength, mental and physical, as it is needed in the activities. When, through the fast, dead and noxious refuse is eliminated, the expression of each of these qualities is evident, and we learn that man does not depend upon food for strength, nor for the accompaniment of energy, body heat. Food is needed only for the repair of broken-down tissue, for the up-building and rebuilding of the framework that carries the human soul. The conclusion is not to be drawn in the absolute that strength will be manifest and that life may be continued indefinitely in the absence of food, nor is it to be assumed that in the process of evolution man may reach an ideal state of foodless existence. These are but hypotheses of idle dreamers. The source of life will possibly always remain an enigma to finite understanding, and its manifestations can do naught but continue to offer opportunity for speculation.

The theory that human energy and body heat are not derived from food ingested was advanced some years ago by Dr. E. H. Dewey, and every application of the fast for the cure of disease adds evidence to corroborate its verity. In the fast, when elimination has progressed to the point that disease is eradicated, the avenues for the expression of energy and vitality permit of the manifestation of strength - strength that was apparently lost on full daily ration when illness began. As previously noted, in disease the liberation of life force is made impossible because of physical obstacles in the paths of expression. As disease vanishes, natural hunger and strength return. Food is not the source of this phenomenon, since the condition results in its absence. The conclusion is forced that Energy is an entity and that the human body is but a vehicle for its manifestation.

Again, in disease, body temperature and pulse may be above or below register. In the fast, when purification is complete, temperature and pulse are restored to normal. Food plays no more part in the accomplishment of this result than it does in the restoration of strength. Each instance of fasting for the cure of disease perfectly demonstrates the basis in fact of the theory that food serves the sole purpose of repair and growth of body tissue, and that the source of vital energy and of body heat lies without the human frame. The brain is its organ of reception, and it is significant that this instrument of function recovers from fatigue through rest and not because of the assimilation of food. Nerve sustenance is obtained from its storehouse in the body, but nerve energy is renewed through the breath of life.

CHAPTER XIV: CHILDREN IN THE FAST

'Keep the young generation in hail and bequeathe them no tumbled house.'

George Meredith

When the human child is born into the world, it is equipped with but three developed faculties hunger, thirst, and sleep. The infant, if capable of expressed desire, would signify its greatest need as sleep, but its rest is naturally punctuated with hunger periods, and at these times and at no others it should be fed. To awaken a quietly sleeping child for the purpose of administering food is most inadvisable, yet nurse and mother, burdened with professional tradition and advice, in overzealous care rarely permit a two-hour interval to pass without forcing food upon the attention of the baby, asleep or awake. The child will, through habit, take the breast and suckle for longer or shorter time, but its rest has been disturbed, and its small digestive apparatus is never free from labor as long as mother or nurse can stimulate appetite. Disobedience to natural law brings its penalty, and disease invariably appears to right the wrong. Feed the baby only at the dictate of the natural hunger cry, but begin the process at the beginning before a vicious habit of expectation and appetite has a chance to form. With the exception of inherited blood taint, overfeeding the child is the great cause of infantile disease, and it could not occur if the first hunger instinct were permitted to guide the infant from birth. Actual need alone would then be satisfied, and the artificial sense of appetite that might develop could be curbed and directed. At birth the physical connection between the child and its mother must of necessity be severed. One of the mistakes in modern obstetrics is the wide-spread practice of cutting the umbilical cord before the cessation of its natural pulsations. Interchange of oxygen and of nutriment between mother and fetus has taken place through this avenue for the whole period of gestation, and by this means alone has the baby frame been built to the moment of birth. Its final use and its last pulsations insure tissue-nourishment sufficient to carry the child until food for post-natal growth can be furnished from the breast of the mother. Nature thus provides for the maintenance of the child-body until the maternal supply is ready to be utilized. Haste in cutting the cord starts the infant badly, and hunger is asserted much earlier in these circumstances.

When departure is made from the laws of nature, abnormal physical conditions are produced, and penalties are exacted. The normal food and the only food that is designed for infant use is mother's milk. At birth delay in its appearance is often noted, and perhaps for two or three days its secretion is absent. Reference to the function performed by the umbilical cord directly after birth offers explanation why, in this event, excessive haste need not occur in attempt at artificial feeding. If, as unfortunately is too often the case in modern life, the mother finds herself incapable of furnishing food for her child, a substitute can then be obtained. The ideal method makes use of the wet-nurse, and, if this cannot be done, water-diluted top-milk from a healthy cow, with sugar of milk or honey added sufficient to supply as nearly as possible the constituents of mother's milk is the nearest and best alter- native. Prepared foods are doubtful in effect, and they agree with the child, or rather the child agrees with any one of the many kinds on the market, only in exceptional circumstances.

The contention that all disease has its origin in impaired digestive power is more strongly upheld when disturbances occur in the young than when the adult organism is affected. In the child, unaccustomed to continued abuse of the body and its functions, and with no harmful habits formed, the system resents any but natural treatment. If the contrary is persistently followed, disease develops.

The physical condition of a nursing mother is invariably reflected in the body of her child, and mental disturbances, temporary or permanent have like effect. Through nervous derangement of functional power, induced by disease or by anxiety, grief, or anger, such changes are occasioned in mother's milk as to cause serious illness in the suckling child. It is therefore incumbent upon the parent so to regulate her physical body through a dietary regime as to correct in herself the error in milk quality, and so to conserve her mental forces as to prevent systemic disease and nerve tension, with their detrimental influences upon infant digestion.

When infantile disease is manifested, a medically treated child is still more hampered in its physical processes. Drugs are poisons, and their introduction into the body of an infant suffering from food excess or from the results of erroneous diet in the mother, works havoc with tender nerves and tissue, horrifying to the mind trained on lines of natural remedy. Drugs aim at the suppression of the symptom and not at the removal of the cause, and many an adult body is compelled to struggle through life handicapped by undeveloped, partially paralyzed mechanism, as the result of dosage in infancy.

The disease symptoms of childhood frequently assume what is known as epidemic form. Contagion and infection depend absolutely upon the physical condition of the system and not upon the germ, always present or introduced from other sources. The care of the parent should be directed toward the preservation of health, with its resistive qualities in the body of the growing child; and, if through carelessness, or ignorance, or accident, this condition may fail of conservation, toward the prompt removal of the soil in which the germ propagates and dies. Germicides merely succeed in destroying the microbe, a process that adds decomposing material to an already fertile and expectant medium. And it is reasonable to assume that a poison powerful enough to kill living organisms within the body is of strength sufficient to deal destruction to cell life itself, and this it also does.

Referring to a former statement concerning the administration of food while high temperature prevails, the question may here be asked: Why put food into a feverish infant body? A roaring fire is x>t ordinarily subdued by adding fuel to the flame, and, until disease made its appearance, the patient was ingesting food, and, in all probability, was stricken with a full stomach. Fever, as a symptom, is caused by absorption into the circulation of the products of excess food rotting in the alimentary canal, and, when additional material for fermentation is forced into this mass, either from above or below, the results are a rise in temperature and more aggravated symptoms. The further question is suggested: Why administer drugs at this time? These are either stimulants or narcotics the former increase the action of the heart and with it the temperature, while the latter reduce nerve transmission. In addition medical treatment usually calls for nutriment at intervals of three to four hours, and food is administered in the natural manner, or, when symptoms of an especially acute nature are present, per rectum. In the body of the child, the effects of both overfeeding and of drugs are long-lasting, and here most emphatically the method to be employed should remove fermenting rubbish, the cause of the condition. As in the adult, when disease appears, prompt withholding of food removes through active elimination the immediate cause of disturbance; an enema, or several of them, cleanses the bowels of toxic digestive products; fever is abated; diarrhea and colic disappear; and in two or three days at most the youngster is again whole and hearty. For children respond to the fasting treatment in marvelous manner; their natural forces have not been depleted by years of excess in physical indulgence, and are present in pristine vigor. No alarm need be felt, since nature readjusts the little system most rapidly, and its functions at once resume their labors refreshed and re-invigorated. A fast until hunger makes its demand is mandatory in even the slightest digestive ailments of the smallest of babes; and a comparison of this method of treatment with that which requires the stomach to be dosed with drugs, and the very blood itself to be permeated and vitiated with the products of disease in lower animals in the forms of virus and serum needs no commentary.

Similarly the enema may be given to the infant, using, of course, an amount of fluid commensurate to the size of the infant bowel, and, if judiciously repeated, the colon is flushed of its poisonous contents, fever subsides, delirium, if present, ceases, and disease vanishes. The enema may be administered to even the day-old babe with beneficial results, for it serves to clear the colon from clogged and thickened secretion, and, when feeding has begun, especially if the milk of the cow or prepared foods are used, the products of their imperfect digestion are at once removed. The ease with which the fretful, colicky babe may be relieved by the careful use of the internal bath is a matter which every mother should understand, and its application at judicious intervals during infancy is of equal importance with its bi-weekly employment in adult life.

Whenever in a young child the slightest evidence of disease makes its appearance, whether in the form of nasal discharge, of constipation, of diarrhea, or of internal pain, it should be considered as ample warning of loss of balance between nutrition and waste. Food should be at once omitted, the enema administered, and treatment continued until equilibrium is restored. If this method of handling the situation be consistently followed, no need will occur for later alarm lest acute disease symptoms or morbid organic structural defects, such as adenoid growths and enlarged tonsils, develop. Care at this time precludes dependence upon the knife of the surgeon in infancy or in adolescence.

Repeating the caution expressed in the first paragraph of the present chapter, freedom from disease in infancy and development of strong resistive qualities in adult life are dependent upon normal feeding in childhood. No food except as hunger dictates. And, further, the child must be permitted, not only to signify its need, but also, after it is weaned from the milk of the mother, to select within reason the kind of food desired.

If no abnormal craving has been developed through forced feeding, or through food other than mother's milk, taste will not have been vitiated, and in its wants the child itself will pursue its natural inclination, the only law upon which health depends. Hands off! Follow nature! Do not attempt to act as her guide!

The moment that disease is recognized in its true character as a natural process of cure, the real and only specific for the child, as for the man, is discovered rest for the overworked organs of the body, and renewal of those functions that need repair.

NOTE: DETAILS OF THE ADMINISTRATION OF THE ENEMA TO THE INFANT!
IMPLEMENTS

The usual fountain syringe, equipped with convenient shut-off and with two small-sized rectal tips.

A low chair, admitting of holding the recumbent child in the lap at a height slightly above the level of the bowl of the toilet.

Two pieces of rubber sheeting, each one yard in length. Throw one piece over the top edge of the raised seat of the toilet, draping it so as to receive spatterings or forcibly ejected discharges from the bowel. Place the other piece of sheeting half over the lap of the operator, permitting its free end to cover the front edge of the toilet bowl with sufficient length dropping over the edge to convey discharges into the receptacle. A folded Turkish towel should be laid over the end of the sheeting on the lap in such position as to raise the buttocks of the child slightly and to prevent contact with the surface of the sheeting.

The operator should sit with her right side next to the bowl of the toilet with the infant lying upon its back across the knees.

Care must be taken in inserting the rubber tip into the anus, and the right hand of the operator should hold it in position while the water is flowing through the tube. Greasing the tip with olive oil or with an antiseptic lubricant prevents undue irritation of the mucus membrane of the orifice. The flow may be regulated by the shut-off or by pinching the soft rubber tube of the syringe with the thumb and forefinger of the left hand.

In small children, during the administration of the full contents of one bag of water, it is not necessary to remove the rectal tip from the anus, since the liquid form of the discharge from the bowels permits ejection around the sides of the tube and avoidance is thus made of repeated insertion with consequent irritation. After the exhaustion of the water in the bag, the tip should be withdrawn, and the extra one mentioned in the equipment, unattached to the hose, should be introduced into the anus. Through it subsequent evacuation will occur the more easily, since the constriction of the muscle of the anus is by this means overcome. Neither pipe should be inserted at greater depth than two inches. At this stage of the operation manipulation should be made of the abdomen, following the ascending colon on the right side from the cecum to the transverse bowel, then across to the left side over the transverse portion to the descending colon, and down the latter to a position corresponding with its extremity and outlet. This is an essential that must not be neglected, since it assists peristaltic action and hastens evacuation. Never less than six or eight quarts of water should be used in giving this enema, and, if extreme discoloration in discharge still persists, even more fluid should be injected. The value of the internal bath depends upon the thoroughness with which easily-absorbed fermenting waste is removed from the colon, and this condition is not satisfied until the discharge returns comparatively colorless.

CHAPTER XV: SEXUAL DISEASE AND THE FAST

'Seldom have you seen one continent that is not abstinent.'

John Hales, *'Golden Remains'*

Just what normal sex desire in both male and female originally signified is somewhat difficult to define, but it is safe to assume that primordial sex relations were limited to the purposes of procreation. The ultimate object of the fast is discovered in the restoration of all physiological functions to a primary condition, and this is effected not only with respect to the processes of digestion, assimilation, and elimination, but to that of the sex instinct as well. While the fast is in progress, sexual desire, whether formerly active to excess or abeyant, is brought to normal, and attention to diet and to right living in the future finds passion controlled and desire subservient in all senses to the will.

In the female during the fast the menses may or may not appear, but, after the fast is completed, the monthly discharge may miss several or more periods. Its temporary cessation should occasion no anxiety, for the menstrual flow is at all times a waste product, and, in pregnancy and after the menopause, its disposal is accomplished through other channels. However, instances have been noted in which the menses have appeared, when food was omitted, at irregular intervals almost viscid in consistency and very offensive in odor. This may be regarded as the result of congestion localized in ovaries and uterus, and as a natural cleansing of a reproductive system clogged with refuse.

With respect to the menstrual discharge, the interesting facts are to be observed that it is of regular recurrence during the bearing period in the females of all mammals; that it is barely perceptible in some; and that in none is it so profuse in quantity as in woman. She is the only female in the animal kingdom that is compelled to undergo a monthly inconvenience of copious flow from the uterus; yet this evidence of function is as natural as breathing, but because of perversion in habit, it has become aggravated in excessive degree. Profuse discharge is the penalty attached by nature to the use of the organs of reproduction for other than legitimate purposes, and it is a perfect demonstration of the universal law of compensation.

In treating disease of the reproductive system in the female, the fast both cleanses and relaxes, relieves congestion and restores tone. From one to three days' abstinence from food will correct excessive menstruation, and, when no mechanical defect is present, relief is obtained within twenty-four hours when the flow is accompanied with pain. In this connection attention is directed to the use of the douche, the warm bath, and the enema, while the discharge is present. Medical opinion to the contrary notwithstanding, all of these hygienic accessories are not only helpful, but are absolutely essential at the time of the monthly period. In all cases thorough cleanliness is imperative if the benefits derived are to prove permanent, and right living in after time is a necessary condition of continued well-being.

The menopause, or change of life, is a period dreaded by all women. There is never any certainty as to the time of its occurrence, nor any means of foretelling the character of its manifestations. Treatment by the fast demonstrates that the menses may be properly regulated, and that assurance as to their normal recurrence is possible when right living is adhered to. Similarly purification of the system at the period of the menopause or before, coupled with proper diet and judicious exercise, will fc permit any woman to pass through this experience without distress, excessive nervousness, or other evil consequences.

The object of the fast is achieved in cleansing functional energic avenues and in resting the vital organs of the body. By virtue of these accomplishments the high function of reproduction is not only benefited, but is also restored almost to original ease in gestation and accouchement. Ordinarily, congested healthy secretion as well as impurities deposited in the organs of reproduction are eliminated through the circulation; but even the excessive and offensive discharge that sometimes is present during the fast may be regarded in the light of an eliminative product evacuated on the line of least resistance.

In fact, unless organic defect exist, ever-present female troubles are unknown to nature when her dictates are accepted and obeyed. The fast and subsequent treatment result in a set of healthy muscles for the support of the organs of reproduction and in healthy secretions for all purposes peculiar to these parts. Judicious general exercise and normal nutrition will maintain the sustaining ligaments in strength, and the generative system cannot fail functionally or structurally if normally used.

The dress of woman is responsible for some of her sex weaknesses, and, without entering into details, it is well to call attention to the garment to which is attributed so much of female woe. The corset has no right nor title in the wardrobe of a healthy, normal woman. Her own bones and muscles shape her form as intended by nature, and any woman, not distorted in framework, may attain perfection of figure by muscular freedom and proper exercise. The restriction of a healthy muscle causes it partially to lose its functioning ability, and habitual restraint and unnatural pressure brought to bear upon the muscles of the trunk result in local congestion and in displacement of special organs. Lungs, liver, and intestines, together with the organs of reproduction, suffer from the constrictive effects of the corset, and lack of nourishment, due to restricted circulation thus produced, causes atrophy of muscular tissue, since the latter is not adequately rebuilt. Energy is likewise impeded in the process of liberation; intestines, unable to function, are filled with food rubbish; and congestion, inflammation, auto-intoxication, and sexual decay ensue. The corset alone succeeds in producing many degenerate, breast-less women, who eventually suffer under the surgeon's knife; who cannot fulfil the natural function of child-bearing; and who, if they by accident reproduce their species, are unable to furnish their young with natural food.

The science of Osteopathy has not as yet recognized the ease and the benefit of manipulation of the uterus and its appendages,' and it is only now and then that an osteopathic physician is discovered who, upon his own initiative, has made known the good that accrues by transcending prescribed methods when occasion demands. Fasting will relieve congestion, while manipulation of the uterus and the ovaries from within and without, and of the region of the Fallopian tubes, assisting in this process, will also mechanically adjust the uterus, and will give tone to the condition of the reproductive apparatus by stimulating circulation.

Sexual disease other than that peculiar to the female may be divided into that which is contracted through sexual intercourse, and that which results from lowered nutrition or is transmitted congenitally.

The first class is represented by the local symptoms of gonorrhea in both sexes, of gleet, stricture, and urethritis in the male, of leucorrhoea and displacement of the womb in the female, etc.

The second class is represented by impotence in the male, barrenness in the female, and the various degrees of the blood taint, syphilis, in both sexes.

In discussing the problem of sexual disorder of any kind and its cure, it is necessary to revert to the primary cause of disease, lowered nutrition resulting from impairment of the digestive process. While cleanliness in the female will, in those symptoms that are merely local in character, undoubtedly minimize the chances of infection by contact, the soil in which the germs of venereal disease flourish is distinctly an eliminative product embodied in the fluids of the reproductive tract. The bacillus of gonorrhea, for instance, transferred to either sex, cannot long exist if the products of elimination are normal in quality, and if cleanliness, especially in the female, is properly observed. The former condition is promptly effected by the fast, and the latter is a matter of ordinary personal care. The irritating symptoms of local venereal infection yield to the treatment in few days, and convalescence brings no supervening annoyance, as expressed in urethral stricture, prostatic congestion, etc.

The taint of syphilis, congenital or acquired, if treated before its characteristic organic lesions have developed, is eradicated with equal success, but with somewhat more difficulty, since this disorder is deeply seated, and, affecting the composition of the blood, partakes of the nature of structural defect in vital organs.

Masturbation, a habit of more widely common practice in both sexes than is generally believed, may have its origin in the curiosity of pubescence stimulated by vicious influences. But its development into habitual form requires a constitutional derangement of the functions of nutrition, and the vice of self-abuse is purely a symptom, not a cause of disease. Digestive ferment, occasioning excitement of the nerve centers controlling the genital organs, or local congestion caused by constriction of the waist, by constipation, or by like means, are the active stimulating agents responsible for lascivious dreams and perverted forms of sex satisfaction.

Disease is a unity. The solitary vice is but a symptom, and the fast, applied for the removal of the cause, restores morbidity to health.

In connection with the effects of the fast and of diet upon sexual development and desire, observation establishes the fact that children fed upon a non-flesh regimen progress sexually in gradual, normal manner to puberty, and exhibit fewer tendencies towards sexual abuse or perversion than do those whose diet includes the various flesh foods. A dietary embodying meat is far more stimulating than one purely vegetable in character, for the reasons adduced in previous discussion.

The ideal to be desired in all life is that of equilibrium. Physical existence without normal sex relation is an unbalanced state, nor can it be implied that this natural function, when not exercised, is changed in purpose and acts as an increment to intellect, as moral reformers would have us believe. Far from, it, since, in the male, the propagating secretion is produced only as it is discharged. And, in the female, monthly production and removal of the ovum indicates renewal of fertile cells. In both sexes constant exhaustion of sex secretion undoubtedly draws upon nervous energy and in this manner affects brain power, but the reverse cannot be true. If so, the bulk of the brains of the world would be in possession of continent celibates. Sex and intellect demand impartial exercise, the former for procreation only, the latter for physical control and spiritual advance.

CHAPTER XVI: DIFFICULTIES IN CONDUCTING THE FAST

'Tasks in hours of insight milled
'May be, through hours of gloom, fulfilled.'

Edwin Arnold

The very simplicity of the fast in its application has proved the most serious obstacle to its general acceptance by both the public and the medical profession. Popular writers have lauded its claims in newspaper and in magazine. Books have been written upon it in the enthusiasm produced by the beneficial effects of personal trial, and cures by fasting have been heralded the world over. The consequences are what might have been foreseen. Regardless of the physiology of the human body and the rationale of the method, and ignorant of the physiological changes that the administration of the fast must involve both in function and in tissue structure, inexperienced hands have undertaken the treatment without guidance or the necessary knowledge of the conditions that may develop, and, in many instances, harm with unmerited adverse criticism of the method has resulted.

If human bodies continued to exist throughout life in the normal state they should possess at birth, when functional disease appeared the application of the fast would prove perfectly easy in all cases. But, through constant wrong living, through chronic abuse of the vital processes, and, more than all else, through the paralyzing effects of drug dosage, the average man has acquired defects in organic structure.

In infancy, when disease develops, a drug is given for the suppression of the symptom. In some cases the children die; in others, the paralysis, the functional ruin, of some portion of the intestinal tract or other organ is caused; in still others, the resistive powers of the infant are such as to permit it to survive despite the dose. In any event no true benefit has been derived, and, since the harm was done during the growing state, retardation of development occurs, and, in future years, disease symptoms may be traced directly to the points affected in infancy. With functional troubles continually recurring, these deficiencies in organism finally cause almost absolute cessation of the processes of elimination.

Careful observation of several thousands of fasting cases makes plain the fact that the fast will perfectly relieve all ailments of a functional character, but that it can never wholly overcome mechanical defects in body organism. However, the fast will uncover the organic condition of the system, and will cause the nature of its deficiencies to be clearly displayed. One whose organs are functionally equal to the requirements of elimination undergoes the treatment with no unusual symptoms. But, when severe and distressing manifestations arise during the period of abstinence from food, it is virtually certain that defects in organism lie within. Post mortem examination of the bodies of patients who have died while the fast was in progress gives proof to this all-important point, and, in these cases, it was further demonstrated that death would have occurred, fasting or feeding.

A drug, with regard to its effects upon the human body, may be said to be any substance which will influence metabolism and the functioning of the organs. According to this definition, foods, especially when of unwholesome quality, even though the quantity be reasonable, may react as a drug upon the system. Food itself, like substances regarded as drugs in the ordinary sense, may then act as a poison to the tissue. In like manner the substances formed in the body from the processes of tissue waste may themselves act as drugs in their effect upon living tissue. This occurs when elimination is inadequate. Hence the auto-toxins, through which tissue resistance, i.e., immunity from disease, is reduced, and the way opened for the large group of so-called infectious maladies.

It cannot fairly be assumed that, upon viewing a body after death in the fast, the lesions that may be present in any organ are due solely to previous drugging. Where two such agencies as disease and drugs have been simultaneously acting upon a patient, it is difficult, in the absence of criteria, to decide whether a specific result is due to one or to the other, or to both. But it is a significant fact that, in every instance of death that has occurred in the fast, as covered by the writer's experience, each of the subjects with but a single exception, had been drugged in early life, and that the effects upon organs, as shown in lack of development, were such as would have resulted from impeded nerve action caused by an active poison; and the preponderance of evidence gathered in these postmortem findings lies on the side of drug paralysis.

The constant use of drugs to suppress disease symptoms in the growing child, not only lowers physical resistance, but also retards the development of its organs, in whole or in part, while bony framework and tissue-structure continue to advance to normal adult dimension. The disparity presented by organs of infantile size enclosed in a body fully matured is bound to cause severe forms of functional trouble that will end in chronic disease, since the undersized organs are not equal to the demands made upon them. The function that is predominant while the fast is in progress is that of elimination, and it is easy to understand that, in a body in which portions of the intestinal tract are under dimension, or in which one or other of the vital organs is mechanically imperfect, the work of ridding the system of accumulated poison is beyond the power of the organism to accomplish. As a consequence, to the degree in which organic defects exist, is determined the severity of the struggle with disease, to use orthodox phraseology. In natural terms, the effort which is being made to cast out gathered impurity is made proportionately more difficult when organic imperfections exist. In the adult body, chronic functional disease or drugs may produce like effects, but here the organs concerned are fully developed, and the results are shown, not in arrested development, but in lesions, or in growths.

Whenever, in the fast or otherwise, because of organs undeveloped or functionally paralyzed, the products of elimination cannot be evacuated through natural channels, reabsorption of waste occurs, and the result is displayed in a general poisoning of the blood supply. This condition is known as auto- intoxication, or, as expressed before, the body is poisoned by its own decomposition. This state gives rise in the subject to manifestations that may become alarming. The brain is affected to the extent of mild delirium, hiccoughs appear, or the patient may sink into stupor. Mechanical means of relief in the forms of the enema and of general massage of the body must be resorted to and plied to the utmost in connection with hot applications to the spine and abdomen. In cases not under careful and experienced guidance the situation related will assuredly prove disastrous, and herein lies one of the dangers of inadvisable and promiscuous fasting at unintelligent hands.

The fast cannot cure disease in a body organically imperfect, but the natural physician may direct its use for short periods in such manner as to ameliorate existing conditions and to restore the patient to comparative health. The real state of the body organism is so perfectly uncovered by abstaining from food that the individual thereafter is enabled to live within the limitations of his organs. When the presence of organic defects of more than ordinary seriousness has been determined, the protracted fast is most inadvisable, for, in this event, it is certain that the avenues of elimination will prove in- adequate to exacted demands.

The intoxication that results from absorption of eliminative products has been said to cause delirium sometimes. This condition, present in the fast at times, gives rise to the contention that protracted abstinence from food occasions insanity in the patient. Nothing can be further from the truth, for, when elimination is successfully accomplished, mentality is at its highest; and, on the other hand, cases of mental aberration due to auto-intoxication from overfeeding are speedily restored when food is denied. In fact, auto-intoxication takes place more often when feeding than when fasting, and the overfed body produces poisons the effects of which upon mentality are more dread and more lasting than those of alcohol itself.

The sole explanation of the presence of toxins in the human body lies in the inability of the eliminative organs to function. They cannot dispose of the refuse in quantity to balance intake. In the fast, when difficulty is encountered in this respect, lack of functional power is indicated, and this is due in most instances to congenital organic defect or to early drug paralysis.

The physician who has had long experience in handling disease as a unity is not concerned in any sense with the presence or absence of the various toxins, nor by the symptoms in evidence, except as indices of the state of functioning of the internal organs. If these organs are in normal condition, excess food may interfere with function through congestion. But the vital parts of the human body are in many instances drug-paralyzed or food-stimulated, and, medically speaking, they are brought into action by the administration of additional drugs or by further food-stimulus. Elimination can then take place only abnormally, with, in all cases, but partial evacuation of body waste. In the natural treatment of disease, the character of the toxin need not be considered, save in so far as it is an indication of the severity of disease, while the thought paramount deals with the condition of the organs rather than with the nature of the circulating poison.

The statement is often made that the fasting patient subsists upon his own body while food is denied. This is absurd, for the dominant process in action at this time is that of elimination of waste, which at no point was available for repair of tissue, and which, stored throughout the system, acted only as an obstacle in the avenues of vitality. This is so even of that part of the refuse that had entered into cell composition, since the presence of disease has made apparent the fact that this matter has been rendered harmful by decomposition through delay or arrest of elimination. The diminution in weight of the body during a fast is due to the removal of waste, and the change in cell life that is taking place must be continued until naught but healthy tissue and tissue nourishment remain. The new body thus created is then ready for the process of rebuilding upon normal lines.

The differentiation between starvation and fasting is made upon the basis that starvation is the consequence of food denied, either by accident or design, to a system clamoring for sustenance, and that fasting consists in intentional abstinence from food by a system diseased and, as a result, non-desirous of sustenance until rested, cleansed, and again ready for the labor of digestion. This might be admitted and yet not alter the fact that the processes in operation are largely identical. But it has been observed that the human body carries a reserve store of nerve sustenance, both in health and in disease; hence, the process of fasting, undertaken only when disease is in evidence, is not at all analogous to that of starvation, which can occur only when the supply of nerve sustenance is exhausted, or, when, as is the case in instances of overfeeding and mal-assimilation, the brain is prevented from utilizing its stored nourishment through obstructed channels of supply. The patient may starve, though well-fed; and in applying the fast, keeping the distinction as stated in mind, starvation begins when the fast ends, or at the return of hunger.

The points of difficulty related heretofore are in a sense technical in character, but there are objections, that at times develop into obstacles, that embody personal opinion and prejudice. In bygone days, when medicine failed to relieve, the sufferer was left without hope, and friends and family prepared for the inevitable. Thoughtful minds, still in the minority, unbiased by tradition, have to-day reverted to nature for help in physical distress, and the natural school of treatment has at last secured itself upon firm foundations. In applying the fast and other natural means of cure, the tendency of tradition-bound intellect is at first to regard these methods as inefficacious because of the absence of nostrum, pill, and plaster. Nothing seems in process of action. The silent and hidden ways of nature, needing no bolus, cannot yet efface impressions trans- mitted through centuries of inherited belief in remedies for the suppression of symptoms. Complete revolution of this idea cannot be hoped for until education on broader lines gives universal independence of thought.

While fasting has been known for ages past as a preventive and a cure for disease, its therapeutic possibilities have never heretofore been scientifically applied. Hence it results that modern employment of the method places the practitioner in such position that no authorities can be consulted, and no personal guidance or advice can be turned to for aid in times of stress. Early years of practice in these circumstances often developed cases in which the patient seemingly declined to the point of death. Family and friends at once condemned the physician and the treatment, and a howling public stood waiting to cry, "starvation," It mattered not that the patient had been given up to die by orthodoxy, nor that the fast had been sought as a last resort. Oftentimes only the sufferer himself was in sympathy with the method, and his condition was aggravated to the last degree by opposition.

A state of affairs such as described induces in a conscientious mind intense concentration on the work in progress. No point that may conduce to favorable issue is overlooked; no natural law or accessory is permitted to remain without investigation. Merely selfish considerations might here prove motives sufficient for earnest endeavor the desire for success, the hope of triumphing over other schools. But a broader, deeper feeling will actuate the true student of nature. In him a perfect under- standing of the law of cause and effect the giving of a truth to the world, the relief of physical suffering are the stimuli that bring success to his work and cause him to surmount the obstacles in his way.

The first discovery of the efficacy of the fast in functional disease was rapidly followed by a knowledge of its value as a diagnostic agent. The method never fails to uncover every weak point in a diseased body, to reveal the exact location of organic distress or defect. Then came the value of proper approach to abstinence through gradual diminution of intake, thus insuring systemic accommodation to the physiological change involved, and permitting elimination naturally to dominate the functions. Here, too, the enema and the bath proved of greatest assistance in disposing of eliminative products.

As elimination proceeds, the observer is permitted to greater or less extent to determine the condition of function of the various organs, and, if mechanical or structural defect is present, it is certain to be detected.

The process of gradual lessening of food supply, in all save acute disease, is the normal rational method to follow first, for the physical reasons given, and second, because of ignorant opposition on the part of the public and the medical profession. Ample time is thus given to discover what is possible under a diet, and the necessity of continuing the treatment by a fast is fortified by the knowledge thus obtained.

When merely functional disease is in question, the case in treatment is simplicity itself, unless dissipation, excessive nervous expenditure, or serious blood taint, has largely prohibited vital expression. Patients of this class are ordinarily able to care for themselves throughout a fast of average length.

Whenever organic disease exists, whether in the form given in Class 2, or that in Class 3 in previous discussion, unpleasant symptoms are bound to arise. And at times all the courage and the wisdom of long experience in handling disease by the method of nature are needed to meet the conditions. Knowledge of the causes of delirium, of stupor, of any and all of the symptoms of toxic poisoning, none of which can be wholly overcome in extreme organic disease, makes faith in the method unshakable. When death occurs, it is inevitable; it cannot come except when it is not possible for the vital organs to function longer. The life of the patient is extended through abstinence from food, since organic effort is thereby greatly reduced.

In the event that grave organic defects exist in a patient, signs, more or less determinant, are expressed in both the time of preparation and in the early days of the fast. Serious symptoms do not usually appear before the third week of abstinence. And then these demonstrations may assume any of the forms of .weakness, even to loss of mental control. In the writer's own experience, four cases are noted in which at this period violent delirium, several days in duration, occurred. Two other patients were for longer time mildly delirious. But all, even those in whom death intervened, emergence from the mental cloud and continued to dissolution or to recovery with perfectly clear mentality. It is in cases such as these that human helplessness is most apparent, and here the lesson is learned that man must cooperate with nature and follow her laws.

In examining a body diseased it is possible to locate by palpation, or feeling with the hand, the lower bowel throughout its extent, by using a copious enema after the intestine has been flushed of its contents. Filling the colon with water rounds it out, and its form and position can then readily be discovered through the walls of the abdomen. In all cases where extreme mental disturbance was noted, the transverse portion of the lower bowel had failed from its normal position to the region of the bladder. In this situation the contents of the small intestine, when discharged into the caecum, were incapable of rapid evacuation, even with the assistance of the enema, and brain congestion followed the extreme condition of auto-intoxication produced by the absorption of the ferment thus created. It has been dwelt upon in the chapter on mental and bodily reaction that physical disease induces mental disturbance. There can be no doubt that many inmates of asylums are curable through the relief of conditions identical with those here described. A regular physician, prominent as an expert on insanity, recently made the following published statement: "For the checking of insanity, the crying need is a study of the causes of the malady with a view to its prevention. Nine-tenths of the inmates of our insane asylums are incurable, according to our present knowledge. What an argument for the prevention of the disease!"

Other instances where organic development of the small intestines has been arrested in early life through disease and drugs, give rise to unpleasant symptoms and require most careful attention, not only in the fast, but in the after period of dieting. These cases never occasion mental crises, however.

The latter are uniformly confined to instances such as cited above.

As has been said, fear, the dread of death by starvation, calls down upon the fasting patient, despite the courage of his convictions, the torture that follows acts in opposition to the wishes of affection. And, often, in sheer hopelessness of family cooperation, and in spite of personal faith and benefit, the fast is abandoned and drugs are again resumed.

In the fast there can be no danger of starvation. The great safeguard of all life is hunger true hunger not appetite. And, when the process of purification is complete, hunger returns and food must be supplied.

Skill in the treatment of disease by natural methods cannot be acquired from books, for there are none in print as yet with detail sufficient to cover all points. Years of experience in applying the method to ailing bodies alone can give the knowledge necessary for overcoming the difficulties that may and do arise. And constant practice and observation of the phenomena of the fast convincingly establish that the beginnings of disease lie at the threshold of digestion. Its seeds are sown in the mouth, while stomach and intestines, injured by food improperly masticated, and worked beyond limit by oversupply, continue and conserve their propagation. Impaired digestion and impure blood are cause and effect.

It cannot be too strongly borne in mind that fasting in itself is but a means to an end, a cleansing and resting process that prepares the human body for right living in future time. A cure cannot be accomplished until the individual, cooperating with nature, completes what the fast began.

CHAPTER XVII: CURES BY FASTING

'There is no chance in results.'

Ralph Waldo Emerson

The cases dealt with in the following chapter are typical but not exhaustive. They are selected from a large number solely because of their representative character, and as evidence that the fast reaches indiscriminately but in like manner all phases of the functional bodily ills, and all organic disease that is not beyond repair. In the first instance the patient was afflicted with the disease symptom known as inflammatory rheumatism. When first seen, the boy, for he was but seventeen years of age, was in a precarious condition. The case had been given up by the medical adviser as hopeless, and a limit of twenty-four hours had been set within which death must occur. In the opinion of the physician the only thing that could be done was to alleviate the excruciating pain with opiates, thus permitting dissolution to take place while the youth was unconscious from their influence. The distracted family, as a last resort, turned to the fasting method of treatment, and a description of the condition of the young man will perhaps throw stronger light upon the contrast that is drawn between the methods of nature and those of man.

The boy had been in bed for five weeks; his body displayed all of the evidences of disease and of the remedies that had been applied. His left arm, wrist, and hand were greatly swollen and painful, as were also both knees and ankles. The face was flushed, the breathing stertorous, the pulse fluttering and irregular, while the body temperature was 105 degrees. In all respects the working foundation was insecure, and the preceding weeks of medical treatment had been worse than wasted from the standpoint of the natural. For two of these weeks the heart action had been stimulated with digitalis and strychnine; food had been forced upon an unwilling stomach as many times daily as the patient could be induced to swallow; and, when pain had become too great to be borne, or, when delirium intervened, codeine and other opiates had been used unsparingly. In addition, within seven days before change of treatment occurred, two quarts of brandy had been poured into this copiously drugged interior. As a result of drugs and of disease, the boy could neither lie down nor sit up, and his position was a painful compromise.

Death seemed imminent, but food was at once withheld, every trace of drugs was removed, and a slight massage treatment was administered in order to equalize the circulation as much as was possible in the circumstances. At the end of a half hour a warm water enema brought away a large quantity of fecal matter from the colon, and, after this local treatment pulse and temperature showed decided downward tendencies, while the patient was resting more quietly and easily than he had in a week.

In acute cases, such as this, drastic measures are imperative, and on the second day vigorous application of massage and enema once more brought temperature and pulse to lower register; consciousness returned; the swelling in the arm was reduced; and the pain had abated. In one week's time the young man was able to lie at full length in bed, and the swelling, except in the ankles, was scarcely perceptible. Natural sleep had returned ere this, and temperature and pulse were but slightly above normal. During this interval two enemas daily had been administered and masses of impacted feces had been removed on each occasion. Bathing of the body twice each day had relieved discomfort, and at the end of the first week tub-baths were begun and proved of great assistance in the final reduction of filthy internal condition by aiding and increasing elimination.

The fast was broken on the eleventh day with a small quantity of tomato broth fed morning and night, and the amount of food was increased as the patient became able to take care of additional supply. Five weeks from the day of the beginning of treatment, the youth was enjoying a walk of several miles daily, and, after its discontinuance, he adhered strictly to the diet and exercise prescribed and rapidly developed a healthy and robust physique.

The second case, a man 61 years of age, was stricken with paralysis of the entire right side, and, after vain search within the domain of medicine, began preparation for a complete fast. The preparatory period covered but ten days, a time too short to accomplish wholly satisfactory results, but at its completion a fast of forty days, which proved eminently successful in its final outcome, was undertaken. Paralysis, as is well understood, is caused directly by blood coagulation in specific localities of the brain tissue. But one course can be recommended to rely upon natural processes to absorb the clot, thus re- moving pressure and releasing nerve force. Constant accumulation of food material in such circumstances simply prolongs conditions that encourage excessive density of the blood, but the fast, without argument, through rest and elimination, causes natural assistance to be utilized in removing obstruction to the passage of nerve force through nerve channels.

The history of the case was such as will be found in every instance when apoplectic conditions are present in any individual. The patient referred to weighed at the time of seizure 214 pounds. Each day of abstinence testified to a loss in avoirdupois, and, at the end of the fast, the latter had been reduced to 174 pounds. Bile in abundance was discharged with the enemas, and at intervals vomiting of the same fluid occurred. The fast was broken by the administration of grape juice and that of oranges. Within a few days food more solid was ingested. It is as well to quote from a personal letter dated after recovery for the subsequent history of the case.

The letter reads: "I was totally incapacitated from actual manual labor of any kind before my fast, and I lived in dread of a second stroke, with a strange, unnatural depression evident upon slight over-exertion. Great drowsiness affected me, and on occasions I would sleep thirty to thirty-six hours, almost without intermission. My mentality was impaired, my eyesight defective, and my speech impeded. My right hand and arm were clumsy and weak, and at this stage all ordinary human aid seemed powerless.

"I began the fast, and, contrary to my expectations, I had no hunger from the third day to the fortieth. To affirm that there was no inconvenience, however, would be untrue, for by every avenue of elimination most offensive impurities were thrown off, and at times these could not have been borne had the object been lost sight of. My weight, before I undertook the fast was 228 pounds, and the girth of my abdomen, 45 inches.

After I had completed the total abstinence period, I weighed 174 pounds, and measured in girth 38 ½ inches. I am cured of my paralysis; my mentality is clear and normal; my entire digestive system is apparently perfect; my vision is better than for years; my hand and arm are strong; I have no dread of a second stroke; I have no sleepy spells; I feel lighter all over; and, when weary, I am quite refreshed and ready for further exertion after a short rest."

A case of the disease symptom known as locomotor-ataxia, complicated with general derangement of the nervous system, occurring in a female of 28 years of age, also offers itself for description. Preparation was undergone for several weeks and a fast of 22 days resulted in the return of hunger and complete restoration to health. The medical history of this case showed obstinate constipation for twenty years, and there were nervous tendencies that had been persistently aggravated. Medical advice had been followed constantly since birth, yet, when first seen, the muscles controlling legs, hands, arms, and face were in constant motion, and no effort of the will could command their action. During the first week of the fast, rapid improvement appeared, so much so that the young woman was able to walk about without any evidence of extraordinary lack of coordination in movement, and by the fourteenth day all muscular signs of nervousness had completely disappeared.

No unusual symptoms developed in this case. The enemas brought away solid matter until the seventeenth day, and thereafter but a small quantity of bilious fluid. Osteopathic manipulation was daily resorted to, and the loss in weight was not remarkable. There were almost no unpleasant symptoms, and for this an outdoor life and an equable disposition and temperament were largely responsible. After a time devoted to judicious exercises, the patient was discharged completely restored to health and with no remaining traces of the nervous disorder of former days. An added benefit was displayed in the fact that, although there had been decided impairment of sight, myopic in character, the patient was able to dispense with lenses six weeks after the beginning of the fast.

The distressing affliction, epilepsy, is a disease symptom that may be traced to the source of all functional disorder, the digestive machinery, and the case of a young woman, 29 years of age, will demonstrate the effect of the fast and its adjuncts upon this disease characteristic. Before entering upon the fast, the patient had tentatively followed a diet, and had noted decided improvement in general health, but no cessation of the attacks peculiar to the disease named. Medical attendance had been continuous for years, and no improvement had resulted; rather the reverse, for the epileptic seizures had increased in number and in severity as time elapsed. At the beginning of the fast the attacks were recurring at intervals of two weeks, and the latest seizure had happened but three days before. For fifty-six days food was denied, and, from the moment of the inception of the fast to this present writing not a single convulsion has occurred, nor any semblance of an attack, while the general health of the patient has been better than at any time of her life.

The fast in this instance is to be noted in several minor ways, one of which is the fact that on each of the fifty-six days the patient walked a distance of at least two miles; another, that on the fortieth day of abstinence a large mass of dead intestinal worms passed from the bowels in the enema. Improvement was constant from the first, but, after the evacuation of these parasites, it was increased most rapidly, and natural hunger asserted itself on the fifty-fifth day. The loss in weight was normal, averaging about three-quarters of a pound a day.

The medical history of the next instance tells of constant treatment for thirty years for the disease symptom known as diffuse psoriasis. At the time that the patient turned to natural methods, the inflamed, bleeding surfaces characteristic of the symptom covered at least one-third of the skin of the body, and were not confined to any particular locality, but appeared indiscriminately on trunk, arms, and legs; while hands, face, and feet were not affected. The sores were exuding blood and serum and were itching intolerably, so much so that in order to exist in anything approaching comfort, local application of mercurial preparations had long been resorted to, to relieve the pain and inconvenience. But these proved only temporary in effect and the symptom returned in a short time more angry and more obstinate.

The general health of the patient was excellent, and to this a strong constitution and a robust physique contributed. Perhaps, as is often the case, the outlet that nature had established in this instance was most salutary in so far as the appearance of other disease symptoms was concerned. This fact is held to be proved in instances of syphilitic infection, for here all outward evidences of disease are invariably subordinated to the direct blood taint.

When first under observation the patient weighed 172 pounds, and her habits were those of a woman in comfortable circumstances with the idea ingrained that three and even four generous meals daily were necessary for the preservation of health and strength. She was, however, discouraged and disheartened because of the intolerable distress occasioned by the state of her body, and, as a last resort, considered what, to her, meant living death, the fast.

After three weeks of preparation, the period of abstinence began, and continued without interruption for 75 days. At no time during this interval was any food ingested and at no time was the patient unable daily to cover on foot the distance from her home to the place of osteopathic manipulation. Undoubtedly this was partly due to her magnificent physical organization, as well as to a will power equal to the attainment of the object in view. As a consequence the case was easy to treat and, with the gradual subsidence of disease, early opposition was conquered by faith in the outcome.

The fast was typical, and was remarkable in nothing save its length. The loss in weight was not unusual, and at the end of the fast but thirty-two pounds had been eliminated, and the patient weighed on this date 140 pounds. Until the twentieth day chilliness and temperature below normal were noted, and, while pulse and temperature remained below register in the early stages, by the sixth week normal register had been reached. The enemas contained solid feces until one-third of the fast had been finished, and thereafter, until the last week of abstinence, large quantities of yellowish-white mucus were discharged. This catarrhal refuse indicated that elimination had been re-established through normal avenues. Up to this point the greater part of internal filth had been cast off through the pores of the skin, an abnormal condition that had directly caused the suppurating areas on the surface of the body.

It was not until the fourth week that visible improvement in the exuding sores became noticeable in any degree. The itching subsided with the cessation of exudation, and the latter began to diminish to an appreciable extent about the end of the third week. From the time mentioned until hunger returned, the inflamed areas rapidly healed, and healthy skin formed in patches that increased and gradually covered the denuded spots.

After breaking the fast, the general health of the patient continued excellent, and the sole remaining signs of former disease were the scarred edges surrounding the areas that were last healed. Even these in time disappeared, and no trace, excepting slight discoloration, which was the result of the previous medical treatment that the case had received, was left as a reminder of the hideous disfigurement of earlier years.

At no time during the long interval without food was any alarm felt concerning the ultimate outcome either by the patient or by her physician. Fear enters and disaster results in cases not properly conducted solely because of ignorance of the physiology and of the philosophy of the fasting method of cure, and the case is but another instance demonstrating the fact that, in the absence of organic imperfection, there is positively no danger in abstaining from food until nature asserts that the elimination of disease is complete.

Another case presents itself that of a woman 34 years old, in which the fast was undertaken for the relief of general disease resulting from years of wrong living and of erroneous treatment. Organically speaking, there was a mechanical defect in the dorsal vertebrae, two of which had been displaced in such manner as to compress the spinal cord thus causing complete paralysis of the lower trunk and legs. The slipping of these vertebrae was directly due to mal-nutrition of the dorsal muscles, and in all her life the patient had never known a moment of health, while intermittently in earlier days severe fevers had occurred, which finally created contractions in the descending colon, a condition that caused constipation and subsequent septicemia. When first examined, the case had been bedridden for one year, and a congestive chill was the immediate severe symptom that indicated the employment of other means than medicine for cure. The fast was entered without preparation, and was carried to a successful end after 58 days.

The medical history of this case showed an inherited tendency towards scrofula, and there had been manifest at intervals offensive running sores, while the thumb and the index finger of the left hand had been amputated because of a non-healing abscess. These ulcers had been, without exception, diagnosed as tubercular in character by previous attending physicians and had been treated from the medical standpoint accordingly.

Two days after the fast began, an abscess, similar in nature to those from which the patient suffered, broke through the surface of the skin at the base of the spine immediately over the sacrum. The discharge from this sore was most profuse and offensive, and the affected area spread until it was at least three inches in diameter, while its depth became such that the periosteum of the sacrum was exposed within ten days after the breaking of the skin. For a week hot fomentations were continuously applied, and the gangrenous tissue was carefully cauterized by focusing the rays of the sun upon the ulcer with an ordinary reading glass. By the tenth day the discharge had ceased to be offensive, and a few days later healthy granulation began. When the fast was complete, at the end of 58 days, the sole evidence of the sore that remained was a circular spot of slightly reddish normal skin of which the subjacent cushion of healthy flesh proclaimed that natural work of repair had progressed despite the absence of food. This is the point of greatest interest and import to be observed in the treatment of this case, when it is remembered that the blood of this woman had possibly been tainted at birth, and had been poisoned and re-poisoned for years by constant additions to accumulated food rubbish. Elimination had never been successfully accomplished in this body, but, once it could proceed undisturbed, nature was able, not only to cast out existing impurity, but also to repair diseased tissue from the store of healthy pabulum husbanded within.

The results of the copious daily enemas were noticeable for their exceeding foulness, and for the large quantity of dark bilious fluid that was evacuated until the thirtieth day of the fast. The loss in weight was not remarkable and amounted to but twenty pounds, and, when it is considered that the patient weighed only 85 pounds at the beginning of the fast, the proportion of loss as given in a later table was well carried out. While the mechanical difficulty referred to was not wholly relieved at the completion of treatment, the general health of the patient was such at this time as to place her well forward on the road to perfect recovery.

In concluding the history of this case, attention is again called to the healing of a scrofular abscess to the point of complete and healthy closure while the fast was in progress.

Another instance is that of a woman of 28 in whom poor nutrition and what is called a bilious temperament had brought about a condition that manifested itself in periodical headaches and in melancholia with a tendency toward mania. But for the care and devotion of an older sister, the patient would have been placed in an asylum long before coming under observation. In fact, it was because the physician last consulted had recommended that she be restrained that her relatives, in despair, resorted to the fast.

Examination showed a pulse continually at 128 and a temperature that varied from above to below normal with no apparent reason. The diet of the patient had consisted largely of meat and its extracts, and this was at once changed to vegetable broths, while the daily enemas were vigorously applied. At first hot towel packs were used upon the spine in order to control the circulation and to steady the fluctuating pulse, but after a short time these were discontinued since heart beat and temperature made constant improvement from the beginning. Dark, foul-smelling discharges that did not cease until the latter part of the fast formed the bulk of the liquid in the returned enemas.

The patient showed extraordinary vitality throughout the entire period of 42 days of abstinence from food, and she daily walked a distance of two miles, underwent osteopathic manipulation, and returned to her home without undue fatigue. Towards the end of treatment she was able and desirous to increase the amount of her exercise, while her mental condition improved from the very beginning of the dieting period. On the thirtieth day of fasting and thereafter the young woman performed her portion of the housework well and cheerfully. Hunger returned on the forty-first day, and the fast was broken on the morning of the forty-third. Two weeks later the sisters sailed for their home abroad, and a letter written by the patient since their arrival shows a mind in every way rational.

The case of a man 47 years old who had been paralyzed on the right side and who had shown signs of insanity is next noted. The medical history exhibited habitual constipation, periodical headaches, and prolonged bilious attacks. A fast without preparation was begun and continued for twenty days with results that showed the paralysis much improved, bowels regular in action, no headaches, and a steady gain in flesh and strength on diet after the fast. Three months later a second fast was begun and continued to successful completion for full forty-one days. The patient daily visited the office for osteopathic manipulation, and constant improvement was apparent from the first. In neither of the two periods of abstinence from food were there any special symptoms to be noted, and the final result embodied complete eradication of .paralysis and of its symptoms, and great improvement in general health. At the beginning of the second period of fasting the patient weighed 105 pounds; two months after its completion he had regained his normal weight of 145 pounds.

Tuberculosis of the lungs is a disease symptom that needs to be uncovered and attacked in its early stages, and the case of a woman of 82 is given to illustrate its progress under the fast. This patient abstained from food for twenty-four days, but preparation, the fast, and the period of diet after the latter was concluded, covered a time of full six months. When first under observation, examination of the sputum showed numbers of bacilli typical of the symptom; both lungs were affected; chills with fever occurred daily in the afternoon; in fact, the case displayed all the signs characteristic of the symptom named. After a liquid diet for several weeks, the fast was undertaken, was continued for twenty-four days, and no unfavorable conditions of any kind developed. From the beginning an excessive discharge of sputum occurred, but this gradually diminished until evidences of the return of hunger appeared, and, at the several periodical examinations made during the time of fasting, general decrease in the number of bacilli was observed. The enemas were constantly charged with bile and with old feces, and these products disappeared only during the last week of the fast. The chills and the fever vanished by the fourteenth day, and, when the sputum was examined on the twenty-second day of abstinence, there was no trace of micro-organisms. General health was marked by constant improvement after the fast was broken.

The treatment of tuberculosis of the lungs by means of the fast, to insure successful issue, must be undertaken before the stage when excessive structural break-down of lung tissue has occurred. If attacked at this time, a cure is assured. Otherwise, the case classes itself with that of advanced organic disease, which, in the light of previous discussion, bars all remedy.

The symptom named in the medical diagnosis of the next case was valvular heart disease, and prognosis assumed that the patient had no hope of recovery. There was great pain in the regions of the heart, stomach, and liver, and at times in the abdomen. The heart missed one beat in every three; and, in view of the seriousness of the condition, the fast was begun without preparation immediately upon coming under observation. Enormous amounts of dark bilious fluid came away with every enema, of which four were administered daily throughout the fast. Excruciating pain and nervous excitement were experienced until the twentieth day, when at least a cupful of gallstones was evacuated. These continued to be passed until the thirtieth day of the fast, which was broken on the thirty-fifth. The weight of the patient at completion was 174 pounds, a reduction of twenty pounds in thirty-five days. In the early part of this fast there was great chilliness, but temperature and pulse reached normal by the twentieth day, the latter missing no beats. Before this the pulse had been at times above, at times below register according to the degree of activity of the circulating poison. From the breaking of the fast all functions became and continued normal; weight was gained gradually, and soon reached 185 pounds; and from the completion of treatment the general health was perfect.

An interesting addendum to this case is the fact that the patient, after strictly following the rules prescribed as to diet, habits, and exercise for at least a year and a half after restoration to health, lapsed and fell into laxness both in eating and in drinking, with the result that, two years subsequent to the first attack, an abscess formed upon the floor of the stomach, and the patient again came under observation and treatment, and underwent a second fast of forty-five days. The condition at this time gave great pain until the ulcer discharged, which was evidenced by the passage of large quantities of clotted blood and pus from the bowels. The patient hovered between life and death for several weeks, but the absence of food prevented irritation, the ulcer healed, and health returned. The application of the fasting method of cure to a condition such as was exhibited in this patient's second siege with disease is so essentially reasonable and so plain in argument that this description of the treatment of an internal ulcer should convince any unbiased mind.

A short description of a fast for chronic digestive disturbance or dyspepsia is presented in the following case, that of a man 45 years of age. The fast itself covered a period of forty-nine days, and from its beginning until the forty-fifth day the patient was unable to rise from bed. At this date the tongue cleared as if by magic; hunger returned and with it strength; and on the forty-ninth day, when the fast was broken, the patient walked a distance of seventeen city blocks with but little fatigue. No un- usual symptoms, excepting the excessive weakness mentioned, developed during abstinence; and, from the breaking of the fast, improvement was constant and permanent.

In another instance the fast was undertaken for the purpose of correcting functional heart disease, coupled with extreme obesity, by a woman 41 years of age, whose weight was 200 pounds. The patient showed no medical history, excepting that she had submitted to an operation some years previous for the disease symptom known as salpingitis. Throughout the fast the patient was able to attend to her home duties and to take a daily walk to and from the office of an osteopathic practitioner, and these acts were easily accomplished during the long fast of sixty-three days. There was but little faster's chilliness, and there were no unusual symptoms, excepting that, at about the period included between the thirtieth and fortieth days, a gain in weight of from two to three pounds daily occurred, after which a gradual decrease continued, as before, until the end of the fast, when weight was reduced to 140 pounds, and heart disturbance had entirely disappeared.

Medical diagnosis of the next case was based upon dark, ill-smelling fecal discharge, and the symptom was deemed an indication of the existence of cancer of the stomach.

The patient, a man 40 years old, was really suffering from a badly congested condition of stomach and upper intestines, and underwent a fast of fifty days with no marked disturbances. His weight was reduced from 145 pounds to 105 pounds, and the subsequent gain in avoirdupois and in strength was normal, with the result that in two months from breaking the fast, he had re- gained the former to the point of balancing the scales at 170.

Without citing individual instances, attention is directed to the ease with which the disease symptom known as appendicitis yields to the fast. The vermiform appendix in the human body is a slender blind sac opening from the caecal portion of the large intestines. It is on an average from three to six inches in length, and of a caliber of that of a lead-pencil. It is found in man and in some of the lower animals, and in a few of the latter it is large and performs a digestive function. In the human body its use is problematical, but it is more than probable that its function is that of stimulating peristalsis, either through the secretion of a lubricant or by mechanical contractions.

In the medical world, radical treatment of this symptom demands immediate operation and removal of the appendix. Observation of numbers of cases leads to the belief that an inflamed appendix is a symptom most rare in occurrence. The modern craze for cutting living flesh is responsible for snap judgment in diagnosis, and gas in the caecum, gall stones, inflammation of the ovary or of the bowel in the ileo-caecal region, all have been mistaken for an inflamed appendix and have occasioned unnecessary operations with serious and perhaps fatal shock.

In the treatment of any intestinal inflammation, appendicitis included, no assistance is needed other than that which complete rest of the digestive tract and constant application of the enema afford. Pain ceases and fever is reduced in every uncomplicated instance by the end of the third day, and the sole necessity for the continuance of the fast is found in seeking perfect results and the general welfare of the patient.

A young man, 23 years of age, offers a case of the insanity of syphilis. The blood taint was acquired by contact, and, when observed and first under treatment, presented what is known as the secondary stage of the disease symptom named. The mental condition of the patient was such that no physical act was under control, and all abnormal tendencies pursued erotic channels. His weight when treatment began was 150 pounds. After low diet and an absolute fast of twenty-eight days, the time of dieting and of the fast having occupied three months, weight was reduced to 67 pounds. There were no unusual symptoms during the period of fasting, but progress toward sanity was daily noticeable, and, at the end of the time mentioned, mental balance was entirely restored, while the blood taint has never since given any evidence that it ever existed.

A young man, 19 years old, who had been led into habits, mental and physical, detrimental to normal development, became, as a result, a victim of the disease symptom, epilepsy. For five years he suffered from the fits characteristic of the malady, recurrent at intervals of from one to two weeks. Medicine had been appealed to in vain, and when the fast was proposed, it was discovered, after careful examination, that the youth was addicted to masturbation, which, in instances of this nature, is more of a symptom than a cause. A condition of low physical tone seems rather to induce a habit of this kind, and the young man was no exception to the rule. For five months a regime of restricted diet and of fasting was pursued. The absolute fast intermittently included in this time occupied a total of sixty days. Symptoms gradually subsided, and the recurrence of the epileptic seizures became reduced to such an extent that, at the end of the second short fast, four weeks intervened between attacks; and, when feeding was permanently resumed, no further seizures were apprehended. The weight of the patient was reduced before disease was eliminated to fifty-eight pounds, but, from the breaking of the fast, a gradual increase took place, and, at the end of dieting, he had regained his normal of 148 pounds.

A woman, 36 years of age, at the end of the third month of pregnancy developed severe bilious symptoms. Vomiting of dark green bile, and a condition verging upon coma demanded immediate action, so the fast was begun and copious enemas were administered twice daily. The latter brought from the bowels dark discharges, which continued with no apparent improvement until the seventeenth day of abstinence. On the fifteenth, sixteenth, and seventeenth days the patient lay in a semi-conscious state, but revived on the morning of the eighteenth, when the bowel passages were almost normal in color. Rapid return to consciousness occurred, and increased strength marked all succeeding days until the twenty-second, when the fast was broken upon fruit juices, and convalescence thereafter proceeded without interruption.

The loss in weight in this case was 22 pounds. Temperature and pulse were continually above individual normal until the latter part of the fast, the former ranging between 95 and 99, and the latter from 80 to 110, although a decided drop in each was observed after the administration of an enema. No return of the nausea of pregnancy occurred after breaking the fast, and thereafter the general health of the patient was excellent. At term an eight-pound child was delivered, perfectly developed and vigorously healthy.

On the fifteenth day of this fast, in view of the gravity of the situation, a consultation was held with a former medical adviser. The latter advocated, as the only means of saving the life of the mother, the immediate removal of the fetus, and the abandonment of the fast. His opinion was overruled, however, and the result of the case fully justified the stand taken. As the officiating physician at the confinement, five months later, he expressed himself concerning the ease of delivery and the remarkable vitality of the infant, and acknowledged his error in judgment by a complete reversal of his condemnation of the fast.

An analogous case is that of a woman of 27, wife of a practicing physician. She was between three and four months pregnant, and was suffering severe pain in the region of the uterus and in that of the stomach. The former organ was found to be displaced. Nausea and vomiting were constantly distressing the patient when the case was presented and the fast decided upon. A preparatory period of twelve days on liquid diet preceded the latter, which continued for thirty days. No unusual symptoms arose during this time, and constant improvement was noted from the beginning, the sensation of nausea decreasing successively and disappearing about the twentieth day with no return thereafter. Pulse and temperature remained slightly below normal until eating was resumed. The fast was introduced and broken upon strained vegetable broths, and solid food was eaten twelve days from the date of its completion. At term the patient was delivered of a babe weighing seven pounds, as physically perfect and as healthy as that described in the previous case. The loss of weight in this fast was an even thirty pounds.

It is to be remarked that the children of these two mothers are not only physically excellent examples, but are also mentally intelligent to a marked degree. These gratifying characteristics are to be attributed to the purification in body undergone by the pregnant women at a stage early enough to provide for cell structure in the forming child unvitiated by disease in the system of the mother.

The statement of the following case is in the language of the father of the patient:

"During several weeks prior to his sixth birthday, our oldest boy had complained of sore throat and general lassitude. This finally developed into an acute tonsilitis. On the third or fourth day he complained of pain in both knees, and by evening these joints were swollen and red, and the pain had become so intense that the weight of the bedclothes was unbearable. The physician whom we called one of the regular school promptly diagnosed the case as one of inflammatory rheumatism. He advised the use of hot applications to subdue the pain, and insisted on putting the left knee, which was the worse, in a splint so that it could not be moved. On his second or third visit he discovered mitral regurgitation, that common and ominous symptom, showing that the systemic poisoning had affected the valves of the heart. His prognosis was most unfavorable. He said that the acute stage would last probably six weeks, and that it would leave the patient with organic heart trouble.

"At this point we decided to resort to a method in which we had long believed, but which we had failed to try at the outset of this sickness because we had not realized the seriousness of the case. We discharged the physician and began the treatment described herein under the direction of a competent natural practitioner. She took off the splint and gave both knees a careful but thorough rubbing. They had been apparently too sensitive to touch before this, but by the time she had finished the massage, the child said that they felt better. She told us not to bother about his heart or anything else in the line of symptoms, but to stop feeding him, to give him daily baths and manipulation and to watch nature do the rest.

"The pain kept up at intervals, intervals which grew steadily longer, however, for two days, then ceased entirely. Before the end of the week, the patient was able to be taken down town on the street car for his osteopathic treatment. His fast lasted twelve days.

"Later in the summer he had a recurrence of an old eye trouble, one resulting from an impure condition of the blood. He had been treated the summer before for this trouble, which had lasted several months. This time we began another fast, which continued for twenty-two days. At its end he stripped the bandage off his eyes one evening and looked at us and we knew that the thing was conquered. During a few of the twenty-two days he had a little orange juice, and at all times he had all the water that he desired. A daily bath and rub were given, and a copious enema each morning and evening.

"At the time of writing, two years from the date of the last fast, there has been no recurrence of either the throat trouble, rheumatism, or eye trouble, and a regular physician, a friend of the family, who examined the boy a few months ago, pronounced his heart perfect."

The next and last case is that of a cancer of the right eyelid of twelve years standing in a man 62 years old. The patient had been twice operated upon without success, and the cancer made its third appearance in most virulent form. A consultation with a medical specialist resulted in renewed recommendation of the knife to which the patient refused to submit. He began preparation for a fast which lasted forty-five days, and at the expiration of this period all that remained of the suppurating sore was a reddish scar of its former seat. Four years later his personal report of the case shows no symptom of recurrence upon the eyelid or elsewhere, and general health superb. The eradication of this symptom of extreme blood impurity by means of the fast fixes the value of the treatment in supposedly incurable forms of disease. It bears out completely the contention that disease is a unity, and that its cure lies in the application of the single method of nature, elimination. Cancer is merely a symptom of general disease, and it may be eradicated when its ravages have not involved an organ to the extent of rendering it incapable of function.

A cancer, a tumor, are evidences of nature's economy in gathering her forces of cure at a single point. Medicine seeks to "drive it in;" surgery to "cut it out;" neither succeeds in removing its cause. Even though the actual growth and its nearby ramifications are extirpated by the knife, nature is still impelled to rid the body of its circulating impurity by constructing destructive cells, and only blood purification can accomplish a cure.

The cases cited in this chapter are described with as little technical language as possible, and are submitted in order to show the variety of symptoms treated, all of which revert to the fundamental principle dwelt upon and emphasized in the text that there is but one symptom of disease, impure blood; and that it has but one cause, impaired digestion; and, further, that any and all of its medically-termed manifestations, because they are results from the same origin, will yield to the remedy indicated and prescribed by nature.

Faster's chilliness, referred to in a number of instances in the text, should not necessarily convey the idea that body temperature in these cases was below normal. At any time chilliness is simply a condition of sensation, and in the fast it is due to the absence of food stimulation, as previously described. Then, too, it is to be recalled that normal pulse and normal temperature are relative terms, and that their limits vary with the individual. In many of the cases quoted and in others not mentioned, temperature was below register during part of the fast, but the application of the treatment and its accessories invariably restored these conditions to normal for the particular patient.

Attention has been drawn to the fact that when death has occurred during the fast, the organic trouble revealed showed in each instance that some paralyzing influence had interfered in early life with the functions and had retarded the development or structurally affected the organs. Original defects thus caused have always been located in the organs of digestion, which displayed con- tractions, accumulations of morbid or of healthy tissue, and lesions that lead to but one conclusion, viz. barring congenital deficiency, these deformities, without shadow of doubt, are caused by powerful drugs with which the science of medicine formerly saturated the system.

A reference to the chapter, "Death in the Fast," will illustrate the lack of development in bodily organs. In several of these cases, degeneration of one or other of the large digestive glands the liver, the spleen, and the pancreas is also revealed. In one particular subject the pancreas had become a mere cartilaginous replica of the original organ, a petrified reminder of its former self. In another case, a hardened ring of muscular material had brought the walls of the stomach to such a state of contraction that distinct and separate pouches were formed, and the floor of the organ at the contraction lay within a half -inch of its upper wall. Contractions existed also throughout the length of the small intestines, but those portions, which were in functional state between, showed conclusively that the organ had fully developed, and had been originally of normal size and function, but had been acted upon by some corrosive agent that had caused the deformation. In other autopsies intestines were of infantile size, and exhibited a condition that made known the fact that at no time after the third or fourth year of infancy had they ever added to their structure or to their capability of function. The cause of this result must also be ascribed directly to the same malignant influence the administration of poisons, of paralyzing extracts, that destroy nerve transmission and occasion paralysis of function and of organ.

It is evident that the word, "science," defined as "to know," cannot be applied to medicine as a curative system for disease. No practitioner is able to foretell the effect of a drug upon successive patients. One may be stimulated, another stupefied, and these results may be reversed when conditions are changed. The physician of the future will forsake symptoms except as indications for local relief, and will devote himself to the prevention of disease, to the Science embodied in the unchanging laws of nature.

While the rest and the purification that result from a completed fast are the basis of the method of treatment, additional means that can in any way assist in attaining results are never neglected, and these material aids need not ever enter the domain of medicine. Osteopathic manipulation, intelligently applied, proves of great value at all times during the fast and thereafter. Chiropractic adjustment of spinal column brings relief and comfort. And each of these schools, with their limitations recognized, are yet to be reckoned as important adjuncts on curative lines. The differences that arise among members of the medical profession are such as cannot occur among those who reason with nature from cause to effect, nor is it necessary for the natural practitioner to wait until disease has reached an acute stage before making diagnosis.

CHAPTER XVIII: DEATH IN THE FAST

'It is hard to take
'The lesson that such deaths mill teach,
'But let no man reject it,
'For it is one that all must learn,
'And is a mighty universal Truth.'

Charles Dickens

Death under medical treatment, in the majority of instances, results from disease that is functional, not organic. In the experience of the writer, death in the fast never has occurred when merely FUNCTIONAL disease was present, and never has resulted from abstinence from food, but was the inevitable consequence of obstruction by ORGANIC imperfection of the avenues through which the energy of the body is expressed. In this chapter medical evidence in cases of death from alleged starvation is compared with first-hand knowledge obtained in applying the fast for the cure of disease, and from post mortem examination of the bodies of patients who died while under treatment.

The immediate cause of the cessation of life is discovered in the fact that the brain becomes unable, through disease or shock, to draw upon its reserve store of sustenance for structural maintenance. Some paralyzing influence prevents nourishment of nerve centers and shuts off the life current. No agent more destructive of both physical and mental functions exists than unreasoning fear, and it plays its part in accidental situations where food is denied, such as mine disasters, shipwrecks, and the like, since here mental suffering affects the physical balance, and the cause of death lies in the conditions of the circumstances, and not in the fact that the body is deprived of food, for, in favorable surroundings, weeks and even months may pass ere death occur from lack of sustenance.

It is questionable whether, in a conscious being not afflicted with organic defect, or not situated so that food cannot be supplied when hunger calls, death has ever resulted from starvation, or, in other words, from the exhaustion of brain food stored in body tissue. No conclusive evidence shows that this has ever happened.

The autopsies that were held upon the bodies of the patients, of whom the causes of death are here described, disclosed in every instance organic disease, the origin of which lay in the earlier years of life. In most of these bodies, arrested development of one or more of the vital organs was found, and in all of them defective intestines displayed cartilaginous structure and malformation that must have required either acute inflammation or continued functional disturbance to produce. These cases cover subjects who had followed orthodox methods until orthodoxy proved of no avail, and who then turned to the fast and its accompaniments. Hence it is certain that erroneous diet, with subsequent lowered nutrition, occurring in the developing period of life and later, together with the baneful effects of drugs administered in the attempt to remedy disease, were responsible for the fatal issue. Nature had endowed each of these patients at birth with normal vitality; each of them had suffered in early life from severe functional disorder; and each, with one exception, had been drug-drenched.

Broadly speaking, there is no drug that is not a poison, stimulating or paralyzing in its effect; and, while harm ensues when drugs are employed for the treatment of disease in mature years, the consequences of applying ordinary medical remedies in infancy and in youth are doubly apparent and appalling. It is only necessary to draw the parallel between the results of administering brandy to a child and to an adult to emphasize this statement. What, then, must follow in the event of repeated dosage for fever, colic, colds, and the varied category of infantile disease? And what are the effects of this treatment upon growing human bodies? Not one of us but has the sacred relics of the day of powdered dried toads to blame for organs functionally disordered, arrested in development, or wholly ruined.

Repeating the distinction:

Starvation is the consequence of food denied, either by accident or design, to a system clamoring for sustenance.

Fasting consists in intentional abstinence from food by a system diseased, and, as a result, non-desirous of sustenance until rested, cleansed, and again ready for the labor of digestion. Then, and not till then, is food supplied. Then, and not till then, does starvation begin. The law of hunger draws the line of demarcation.

It may be repeated that, in functional disease, the fast can be carried to its logical end without a, particle of anxiety, because the law of hunger marks the limit beyond which abstinence cannot continue lest the body die. Hence, death from starvation is impossible in a fast properly applied, when it is conducted for the cure of disease not organic. Hunger must return, and food must be supplied. The result in the presence of structural defect is not assured. When the latter is of slight degree, repair is possible and recovery will follow; but, when the faults are such that functioning of one or more organs is prevented, no hope of cure exists, although, by lessening the strain upon other vital parts, life may be prolonged and distress relieved.

Eleven instances of death occurring while the fast or a course of diet was in progress are quoted because of the light they cast upon the diagnosis of disease when natural methods are applied, and because of the exposition made by the autopsies of the effects of erroneous diet and of drug treatment upon the human body. In each case it is shown conclusively that the cause of death was organic disease beyond repair, and that, at the stage reached when the fast was undertaken, no means of cure could have brought about recovery. Two of the deaths described occurred while the patients were dieting, not fasting, but the conditions in these show no contrast, excepting in respect to food or its omission. Death was certain, fasting or feeding. This list of eleven deaths is selected from a total of eighteen, the latter figure comprising all the fatalities of sixteen years of the practice of fasting for the cure of disease. The number of cases treated during this time reaches nearly two thousand, five hundred, each of whom fasted continuously for periods varying in duration from eight to seventy-five days. The death rate is thus seen to be about seven-tenths of one percent.

CASE 1. A married woman, 38 years of age, who had devoted twenty years of her life in vain attempt to enjoy normal existence under medical treatment, finally ascertained that periods of dieting and of abstinence from food were the only means whereby she could obtain relief. At consultation a perilous condition indicating the presence of organic disease was evident, and careful dieting and the employment of the hygienic accompaniments of the treatment were prescribed and continued until six months later. At this time the patient, with full realization of the gratifying relief that invariably appears in disease when organic labor is lessened by judiciously lowered diet or by abstinence from food, and, although advised of doubtful issue, insisted upon entering a complete fast.

After three weeks of gradual reduction in food quantity, the total abstinence stage was reached, and greater relief was at once experienced. On the twentieth day of the fast the patient decided for herself that the stomach could once more tolerate food. Observation demonstrates that patients who have suffered for many years from chronic functional troubles or from organic disease, and who are constantly hoping for cure, have developed, as a consequence of repeated disappointment, a disposition stubborn and willful. They instinctively distrust the hand that may prove the means of recovery, and it is a question whether the better policy lies in acquiescence or in resistance to their expressed desires. In this instance no opposition was offered to the demand for food, and vegetable broths were given. The organs of digestion, as was plainly evident to the trained mind, could not have reached the cleansed and rested state that would permit them to resume their labors, and the administration of food resulted in nausea with vomiting, outward symptoms of organic inability to handle even the small amount ingested. Hiccoughs in severe form, a sign most apprehensive in character and usually indicative of intestinal obstruction, were also in evidence, and continued persistently at intervals until death intervened.

When a case such as this exhibits the symptoms noted in aggravated form, and when, moreover, its history shows years of constant suffering, it is a virtual certainty that organic defects exist that can in no wise be overcome. But, to allay the anxiety of the members of the family, the condition of the patient was brought to the attention of several medical practitioners, who could suggest nothing, for the stomach rejected nourishment, and great difficulty was experienced even in the retention of water. This state continued for more than two weeks, with pulse and temperature at average normal, but with no material improvement. As a final resort, a consultation of medical men was called. Their unanimous diagnosis, based upon the color of the bowel discharges, named the disease symptom as cancer, and the outcome of the case was by them also pronounced hopeless. Inaccuracy in medical judgment is well exemplified by comparison of this diagnosis with the findings of the post mortem examination which followed. Death came at the end of the fortieth day of abstinence from food.

The autopsy made known a condition that the symptoms had predicted. The stomach occupied a position in the abdominal cavity such that its pyloric opening was turned forward and downward six or seven inches; the lower surface of the organ lay opposite the navel, and its normal shape was enlarged and distorted to a capacity of six fluid quarts and to a length of nearly two feet. The small intestines at numerous points were adherent to the walls of the peritoneum, and the stomach itself had to be cut from the same surface in order to expose its whole extent. The medical history of this case notes an attack of typhoid fever, complicated with peritonitis, about twelve years before death. This undoubtedly determines the date of the visceral adhesions, and, in all probability, that of the distortions in stomach and intestines. In attempting to overcome conditions, the gall bladder had enlarged to the size of a pint measure, while the liver was utterly disintegrated.

In the abnormal physical existence of this woman medicine had rendered no assistance, but rather the reverse, and as years passed, disease grew greater. Before the fast, bilious discharges and weakened heart action were symptoms that never varied except to increase in intensity. The fast disclosed from its first day immense quantities of vile, black filth that had been stored within the body, with the result that, from its beginning until just before death, the case showed decided relief and lessened pain. There was, however, no decrease in the amount of waste revealed at each application of the enema, and finally nature indicated that organic trouble defying repair existed, and that death was inevitable.

At the time when typhoid symptoms appeared, all of the organs of the body of this patient had fully matured, but the treatment of the fever and inflammation with drugs, while feeding was in constant progress, led to the formation of the organic lesions described, to which is directly traceable the fatal issue of the case.

CASE 2 is that of a married woman, 39 years old, who had been a sufferer from disease for all of the adult period of life, and who had subsisted upon a diet of liquids for two years previous to death. Since girlhood, she had been treated without drugs (which she refused) by many different physicians for stomach derangement, but without success. Her condition grew worse month by month, until, in sheer despair, the fast was invoked, and, while death occurred at the end of fifty-seven days, the relief experienced leads to the expressed opinion that the treatment prolonged life for some weeks.

When the body was examined after death, the condition revealed was this: In the duodenum, just below the pyloric opening of the stomach, there must at one time have existed an ulcer or acute inflammation. Nature in her efforts at repair had deposited tissue cells at this point to the degree that the entire lumen of the intestine had finally been obstructed with the growth. There was no evidence of the characteristic cell formation of cancer, but merely that of an accumulation of tissue that occluded the gut. The right kidney was in a state of complete disintegration, but the other organs, and the intestines throughout, with the exception of the portion named, were normal in size and position. Until a year or more preceding death there may have been a small passage through the growth described, but this had finally closed, and the woman had lived only by the absorption of such liquid food as she could ingest and retain. The condition of the major portion of the intestines as to size and position is affirmative proof that the patient had never been subjected to drug dosage in the developing period of life. In this respect this case cannot parallel the one first cited, for in it drugs had played a disastrous part, and were the direct cause of the deformation of the digestive tract. Here the defect was occasioned by natural processes operating for local repair.

CASE 3. A young married woman of 24 had been since maturity a sufferer from severe intestinal troubles, and from acute bilious symptoms. She had been medically treated for so-called appendicitis four years before her death, and an operation had been advised, but to this she refused to submit. In this connection it is interesting to note that the autopsy on this body disclosed an appendix in normal state, with no signs of former inflammation.

Eight months before death the patient had undergone a fast of twenty-eight days and had convalesced into the most satisfactory physical condition that she had known since childhood. During the time of this fast and thereafter she cared for a young baby, and continued to do so until acute bilious derangement, accompanied by symptoms of organic disease, was manifested. The case fasted until death an even sixty days, and it was found, after a few weeks of abstinence, that pregnancy of several months added somewhat to the complications that arose. From the beginning of the fast excessively foul black discharges came away with the enemas, and there was a constant, slight daily rise in temperature, which, however, was invariably reduced to average normal after the administration of the internal bath.

At the post mortem examination it was discovered that the liver was in a condition of complete disintegration; the stomach exhibited an extreme hour-glass contraction, and its pyloric opening would not permit the insertion of a lead pencil, nor could it be stretched without tearing, on account of the hardened nature of its walls; the small intestines and the colon throughout their length displayed a series of cartilaginous contractions. In this instance these contractions were formed after full development to adult life had taken place. They undoubtedly were the results of powerful drugs administered from time to time after the eighteenth year, since all other portions of the intestines were of normal size. The fetus was removed from the uterus at the autopsy and was found to be in perfect condition, exhibiting the normal development of an unborn child of four months.

CASE 4, that of a married woman of 85, was similar in many respects to the one preceding. This patient fasted fifty-nine days from the beginning of illness until death, and the case was complicated with an extra-uterine pregnancy in the right Fallopian tube, which aggravated conditions until the fetus was prematurely delivered. The whole adult life of this woman had been made wretched by digestive disturbance, bilious attacks, and menstrual difficulties. Drugs and patent medicines had done their worst until two years before death, when, in hopeless apathy, the patient consented to undergo a fast, and completed one of thirty days with such success that she experienced entire relief from the menstrual pain thereafter, and had no digestive distress unless careless in diet.

The cause that compelled the patient to enter a second fast lay in organic disease that had progressed to the point that the functions became inoperative. Disintegration of the liver must have existed for some time previous to the beginning of the fast, for from its first day large amounts of black bilious discharge came away in the enemas. The condition gradually became so aggravated that the thought of food was nauseating, and its odor and even the perfume of flowers could not be borne. This was also true of the second case cited. Organic defect existed when the former fast took place, and its symptoms were present at that time, but the organs, recuperated by their enforced rest, were enabled to continue partial functioning for some months longer.

In this second fast pulse and temperature rose above normal several beats and degrees each day between the administrations of the enema, but invariably fell to register after the internal bath, which was given twice daily. The fact of an extra-uterine pregnancy having been determined about the third week of the fast, it was discovered on the forty-first day that contractions of the uterus were occurring; the os was dilated, and it was evident that an attempt was in progress to deliver the forming child through natural channels. By outside and inside manipulation of the uterus, a dead, misshapen fetus was finally removed with little or no pain. General relief was instantaneous, and was of such nature as to offer hope of ultimate recovery, but it lasted only a few days, when a decline set in that ended in death on the fifty-ninth day from the beginning of the fast.

Hiccoughs in mild form were present at times during the latter days of fasting, and there was some vomiting of black bile. It was useless to attempt feeding at any stage, for, from the first, the stomach rejected food and water, and the only fluid that the body received during the period named was obtained from the internal and external baths.

The post mortem findings follow: The liver was in such a state of disintegration that even the slightest functioning could not have occurred for months. The gall cyst was at least four times its normal size and contained black bilious fluid. The kidneys were hypertrophied and pocketed with pus. The pancreas likewise was hypertrophied and was so hardened in texture as to resist the knife. The spleen was disintegrated to the extent that it was held together merely by its surrounding membrane. The small intestines were normal in size and position, as was the colon, excepting the transverse portion of the latter, which had dropped below the navel and was no larger in diameter than an adult thumb. The right ovary contained a cyst filled with serous fluid, and the right Fallopian tube was bent twice upon itself. The left ovary was in a state of atrophy and was no larger than a lima bean. The heart and the lungs were normal.

CASE 5 is that of a man of 24 who had been syphilitically infected five years before his death, and had treated the symptoms medically and with advertised nostrums. At the time of consultation the syphilitic sores still remained, and there were other evidences of the ravages of the blood taint present as well. Among the latter was a loss of mental control that compelled the family of the patient to employ a keeper for the youth. About six months before death a fast of twenty-eight days was undertaken and successfully accomplished. The syphilitic sores were completely eradicated at its completion, and relief in general was such that the patient was enabled to dispense with his attendant and thereafter cared for himself. But some months later the signs of organic disease, including loss of mental control, again became apparent. From this time there was a copious discharge of watery mucus from the nasal passages and throat, and a constant, profuse exudation of sweat about the face and the head. The latter symptom was present in such degree that the hair of the patient dripped moisture continuously and his pillow needed changing every hour. Quantities of solid feces and of catarrhal mucus appeared in the enemas, and for a month before death speech was impossible and no function could be performed without assistance. During the last nineteen days of life no food was ingested. The post mortem findings showed a brain, the right hemisphere of which was softened and pus-laden. The left hemisphere was structurally normal. The right jugular vein was filled with a whitish hardened mineral deposit, but the heart was in normal condition. The right lung had atrophied and was in a state of embolism; it was virtually a solid mass of blood clots and was useless as an organ. The left lung was normal. The liver was partially disintegrated. In this case no abnormality existed in the entire length of the alimentary canal, and the kidneys, the pancreas, and the spleen were in functioning condition.

CASE 6, that of a man 46 years of age, presents a physical history of intermittent suffering. As the result of an accident in childhood, in which the patient was internally injured, both youth and early manhood were filled with a succession of acute illnesses, which were treated in orthodox manner with- out permanent alleviation. About fifteen years before death, the patient abandoned medicine and turned to the natural or drugless method of cure, with the outcome that the first physical relief of permanence was obtained. Three years before his last illness acute disease again appeared, and, because of peculiar circumstances, medical treatment was resorted to for a short time but without benefit. Reverted to finally, the fast and its accompaniments succeeded in relieving conditions to such degree that in fourteen days the patient was able to resume the practice of his profession. Although suffering at intervals from that time on, there was no return of acute symptoms until the month preceding death, when, after unwonted physical exercise, followed by a heavy meal, severe pains in the intestines developed. The stomach rejected food; within a week drinking of water brought on nausea; and the point was soon reached when any attempt at the administration of sustenance occasioned excruciating pain. This condition continued for thirty days, at the end of which death occurred.

The post mortem examination showed most abnormal characteristics in the vital organs. The lungs were adherent at every point to the walls of the pleural cavity and to the diaphragm. The heart was in fair condition. The stomach was dilated and prolapsed. The gall bladder exhibited three distinct pouches, any one of which was the size of a normal sac, and two of these sections were filled with one hundred and twenty-six stones, one measuring four inches in circumference. The small intestines were collapsed to the pelvis and were intussuscepted midway in their lower portion so that two yards of their length were telescoped into five inches, and this part measured in diameter of lumen only one-quarter inch. All of the small intestines were below normal in size; the transverse colon lay in front of the descending bowel, an abnormality which largely increased the labor of disposing of body waste; the ascending and descending portions of the colon showed lack of development and were cartilaginous in structure; the sigmoid bend and the rectum were of diameter not to exceed that of an adult thumb, and were also in advanced cartilaginous state; the kidneys, the liver, the pancreas, and the spleen were all in a condition of partial atrophy; the brain and the nerve centers showed no deterioration.

An excuse for surgical intervention sometimes exists, and here was a case in which a condition requiring internal adjustment was presented at the time of the accident noted in its history. Neglected then, life was prolonged by nature in spite of the handicap of physical defect, but at cost of constant suffering.

CASE 7, that of a man 56 years of age, exhibits a history of continuous disease in youth, but includes at least twenty years of later life devoted to diet, to the fast, and to hygienic attention to the body. In fact this part of the man's existence was distinguished by work along all lines of progressive thought. At the time that the case was presented, the patient was aware that, despite all efforts at conservation of health, his condition was such that he must have recourse to every means of assistance that nature could suggest, or he must succumb to the Inevitable. After examination, with the discovery that the symptoms showed marked organic disturbance, it was agreed that but one hope of recovery remained, and that this lay in a complete fast. By it would be determined either the ability of the vital organs to continue functioning, or the assurance that the human machine had reached a point where life could be no longer maintained.

The fast began, and there was no marked disturbance until the twenty-first day, while relief was such that the patient regarded his case as one that showed constant and permanent improvement; but, after this date and during the succeeding ten days, the symptoms became unfavorable, and upon the thirty-second day he sank into a comatose state in which he lay until by manipulation an abscess in the nasal cavity was with difficulty discharged. This release of foul pus eased the patient; he became conscious and assisted with interest in the efforts being made to promote his recovery.

This case fasted thirty-eight days until death. At all times large amounts of mucus were discharged from the colon in the enemas, while pain, sometimes of an excruciating character, was felt in the region of the bladder. In the later stages of the fast and just before death, pus in abundance was present in the urine, and in the last few days of life the urinary organs were utterly unable to evacuate the contents of the bladder, for which purpose an irrigating bougie had to be employed. In spite of the quantity of refuse stored within this body, muscular strength was exhibited in remarkable degree during the fast and until the day of death. The patient was able at all times to move himself in bed, to rise at intervals, and to help himself in ways that seemed marvelous when his physical condition was considered. The results of the autopsy follow: The brain, weighing forty-eight and one-half ounces, filled the entire cavity of the skull, and was perfect in structure. These facts add corroborative evidence to the truth of the theory advanced by Dr. E. H. Dewey, and developed by all who have -given time and practical thought to the treatment of disease by the fast, viz., that, in a fast, nerve tissue is never depleted since its supply of nourishment is gained directly from body reserve and not from food ingested. The lungs were in excellent condition; the heart, organically speaking, was perfect, but was filled with a gelatinous mass of serum affected by post mortem change; from the cardiac opening of the stomach to within two inches of the pylorus there was not one particle of healthy muscular tissue, and the appearance of the walls of the organ was that of smooth, wet chamois skin; the duodenum was below normal in size, but the upper portion of the jejunum was considerably dilated; about midway in the tube of the small intestine a downward intussusception had taken place, in length about two and one-half inches; this was of long-standing, since the walls of the bowel had become cartilaginous and thickened, and in so doing had closed the opening of the gut so that it would have been difficult to insert a lead pencil into the passage; the only section of the colon that was in a natural state was the cecum, but thence to the rectum the organ was of infantile proportion; in fact, there was not one inch of this part of the bowel into which the end of an index finger could have been introduced; the sigmoid flexure was less developed than any other portion of the gut; its bent form was absent, and it had become merely a straight, vertical canal continuing the descending colon to the anus; the liver was badly congested, with its left lobe partially cirrhosed, but its functions had probably been performed with better success than those of the other digestive organs; the gall bladder was distended with bile; the pancreas was extremely small, and the spleen was that of an infant; the kidneys were disintegrated and pocketed with pus, which discharged through the ureters into an inflamed and congested bladder; the latter was very undeveloped and held within its thickened walls barely three ounces of liquid.

The conditions recited were not the results of a fast of thirty-eight days, but were those of disease and subsequent arrested development in early life. While there may have been a lack of general physical growth in the individual, some paralyzing agent introduced from without was responsible for the marked deformity found in the intestines.

In view of the undeveloped and mechanically inadequate state of the digestive tract, it is interesting to record that the sexual organs of this man were those of a boy. He was under height and boyish in appearance as well. Nervous shock presumably received through drugs administered in infancy caused functional paralysis and arrested growth of the digestive organs, and general development suffered in consequence.

CASE 8, that of a young man of 22, suffered for the greater part of his life from acute indigestion attended with distressing symptoms of an apoplectic kind. From the beginning of the fast the enemas brought away merely colored water, but general relief was felt until the twentieth day of abstinence. Then a profuse hemorrhage from the nose occurred, indicating obstructed circulation, and, after the twenty-second day, the patient kept his bed with nose-bleed and hiccoughs intermittently present. At this stage of the treatment the latter symptom in severe form is conclusive of organic defect, and three days before death, when the hiccoughing had become continuous, the patient sank into coma and never regained consciousness. He died forty-nine days from the beginning of the fast.

From the twenty-first day quantities of black bile were vomited, which, as are hiccoughs, is a sign that intestinal obstruction exists, and this diagnosis was completely corroborated by the autopsy. Ten feet of the upper portion of the small intestine proved to have been arrested in growth in childhood, and the walls of the organ were of cartilaginous nature. In the duodenum was discovered an accumulation of hard tissue, similar to that described in CASE 2, which entirely closed the bowel. No food material could possibly have passed this point for months previous to the fast. The presence of this abnormal formation explains two facts observed in the case: the first, that the patient had been compelled to subsist for a year before his last illness upon liquids alone; the second, the absence of solid particles in the returned fluid of the enemas. Repair of body tissue had been accomplished but imperfectly by absorption through stomach walls and those of the short length of upper intestine that might have functioned. The colon at both bends was contracted so that it was barely possible to insert a finger into the lumen, and the right bend had adhered to the transverse portion of the organ in such manner as to form a loop. The kidneys were greatly congested; the gall cyst was much enlarged; the pancreas and the spleen were, however, normal; adhesions of both upper and lower bowels to the walls of the peritoneal cavity had formed at frequent intervals.

In tracing the medical history of the case, it was later discovered that, at seven years of age, a severe fever accompanied by inflammation of the intestines had been treated medically with opiates, and the heart action, as is usual in cases of this nature, had been stimulated to the highest degree with strychnine and digitalis.

CASE 9, a civil engineer, 27 years of age, had suffered since childhood with acute digestive ailments, which were treated as is usual in orthodoxy. Malnutrition finally became so pronounced that the subject decided that medicine could suggest nothing that would alleviate the condition, and he entered a fast of his own volition, coming for consultation some days after its beginning. He died at the end of twenty-one days of abstinence from food. In the state in which this patient was at the first examination, the uselessness of attempting to cope with the organic symptoms that were plainly apparent was so certain that it was deemed best to inform him that recovery was out of the question. Food was administered at this point, but the stomach was unable to retain it, and repeated trials at feeding met with the same result. The fast was perforce continued, and death came, as stated, after twenty-one days.

The post mortem examination revealed an interior with heart, lungs, and digestive organs so extremely arrested in development that, had it not been for the adult body in which they were enclosed, they would have been taken for the organs of a child four years of age. If comment is needed upon this remarkable combination of a mature body with infantile instruments of function, it should be based upon the causes of the lack of structural growth noted. And again the conclusion is forced that, in disease drug-treated in early life, lies the solution.

CASE 10, a man of 34, whose physical history had been one of constant illness after the twentieth year, is next presented. The patient had been treated medically for indigestion, constipation, and various fevers. All his life he had been an inveterate user of strong tea, and in later years fermentation, gas, difficulty in breathing, and abdominal pain invariably succeeded the ingestion of a meal. For the relief of these symptoms medical correctives and tonics were taken but the conditions gradually grew worse. The patient finally decided upon a fast, but, because of family interference, a liquid diet was substituted and continued for thirty-five days, when death occurred. In this case pulse and temperature before the fast had been habitually below normal, and they made but little change during the period before death, the former remaining at fifty-four or thereabouts, and the latter so low that it could not be registered on the ordinary clinical thermometer. There was constant feeling of chilliness.

The autopsy discovered the lungs completely filled with an exudation of serous fluid, a condition comparable to that in croupous pneumonia, and one that was the immediate cause of death. The body, for several weeks, had been blotched or sinused beneath the surface of the skin, the dilated veins showing a circulation obstructed, presumably in the liver. This symptom is always present in cases of cirrhosis or hardening of the liver, and the latter organ on examination was found in an advanced stage of atrophic cirrhosis. The stomach held but eight fluid ounces, and it could hold no more, for its outside muscular coat was in a permanent state of contraction, and the mucus coats were very much thickened, making the whole organ at least one inch in depth of wall. As a result of the contraction of the outside coating of the stomach it had become elongated into a tube, and its normal capacity was much diminished. The duodenum and the upper three feet of the small intestine were dilated so that the lumen was three inches in diameter, a structural change which suggests the thought that nature had attempted to remedy in this portion of the alimentary canal the deficiency in size and function existing in the stomach. It is said that cirrhosis of the stomach is a very rare symptom in disease, but in this case and in the one that follows, this organic change was present in forms that could scarcely have been more perfect examples of their kind. Below the dilated section of the intestines the bowels, including the colon, were apparently normal. The gall bladder was quite small, while the kidneys, the pancreas, and the spleen all exhibited incipient hardening of tissue.

CASE 11, an unmarried woman of 38, had never passed a year during infancy and girlhood free from acute illness, and had been a sufferer for all of later life from nervous exhaustion that at frequent intervals took the form of morbid craving for food, which had been greatly increased when her medical adviser, about five years before death, prescribed its satisfaction by ordering her sustenance every two hours, with a meal the last thing at night. Excruciating pain at the menstrual period compelled the patient for many years to lose four or five days from her duties each month, and left her prostrate and nervous for much of her other time. She had sought the world over for relief, and had turned to the fast and to general natural means two years before consultation, but had undergone only one fast of ten days. Upon examination there was no question that organic disease was present, and, because it existed in aggravated form and no encouragement could be offered in prognosis, it was agreed that the treatment given should be aimed solely at the relief that a light diet would be certain to afford. This course was accordingly pursued and the patient continued upon it for a period of eighty days when death occurred. In this case a sinused condition of the skin of the face and body was noted when first seen; the cheeks were blue and veined, as was also the nose, and the whole body showed deplorable deficiency in venous circulation. This state improved to some extent after entering upon the diet prescribed, but it was never wholly corrected. The examination of the body after death revealed a liver and stomach cirrhosed in structure, and the stomach walls, in addition, showed no evidence of glandular function, their surface being without corrugation, the mucosa having thickened as in the preceding case. The stomach was functionally useless, and its walls were three-quarters of an inch in thickness. The small intestines, infantile in size, were cartilaginous in sections, and adhesions occurred at frequent points. The colon was no larger than an adult thumb throughout, and also exhibited adhesions in various places. The only organs of the body that were in anything like a condition of functional activity were the lungs and the heart. The kidneys, the spleen, and the pancreas, as in the previous case, were incipiently hardened.

It has been mentioned in several of the cases quoted that the patient, after beginning the fast, experienced a renewal of vitality for which no solid physical foundation existed. This was true to a degree in each of the other cases, and was so marked at times that there was hope of ultimate recovery. Nature, struggling to restore organic function, makes the effort commensurate with the gravity of the existent defect. By 'the removal of the labor of digestion at least one-half of the total organic work of the body ceases, and relief that simulates recuperation is manifested despite structural deficiency in the machine. These favorable symptoms continue until elimination of refuse is well under way and proves a task beyond the organs to accomplish when decline begins and progresses until nerve centers and brain can no longer receive adequate support, and the body dies. In Cases 3 and 4 the relief experienced after the first fast in each case was sufficient, with organs still partially able to function, to enable the system to maintain itself until accumulation again became too great to permit of balance. The defects in structure, too serious to have been corrected in the earlier treatment or in the interim, now reached the stage of disintegration or of atrophy, and the liberation of the life principle was no longer possible.

At the time of consultation the presence of serious organic defect cannot always be determined, but no doubt is permitted shortly after the fast begins, for within a week or ten days symptoms are displayed that fix conditions as they exist. The third week positively decides the outcome. In the two cases last described the signs of organic disease were such as not to be mistaken from the first. The result in each instance must be death, and all that could be done to aid possible recovery would, in the circumstances, prove of no avail. Because of family anxiety and the hopelessness of cure, these cases were placed upon restricted diet, a diet that put no undue strain upon the failing functions, but that, nevertheless, did not ameliorate the distress of disease as an absolute fast would have done. Life was prolonged for several weeks in these instances, but, if food had been entirely omitted, relief would have been greater, and days would have been added to existence.

The passing of the life of a human body in cases that are medically treated, in the majority of instances, happens under the influence of opiates that deaden pain and paralyze consciousness. In the fast the end of a life occurs as a quiet sleep, painless, peaceful, and beautiful.

Disease is self-limited; the amount of poison manufactured is determined by the intake of food or of drugs, and eradication of disease is fixed in limit of time by the ability of the vital organs to cast out toxic products. The possibility always exists that these organs may prove unequal to their work, and this possibility becomes a certainty, with death as the outcome, in two situations one, when the organs themselves are structurally defective, and the other, when their powers are stimulated through food or through drugs, or both, to the point of exhaustion. Only one of these conditions, that of organic defect presents itself in treating disease by means of the fast. Both are met in the therapeutics of medicine.

The results displayed in the post mortem findings cited, and the comparisons made in the statement that follows, are tangible assets in the claim that, in the absence of defects in the organs of the body, abstinence from food, with other natural health-giving and health-preserving accompaniments, is the unfailing remedy for the cure of functional ills. The physician and the patient from the outset of the treatment possess the assurance of recovery; and confidence that rests on infallible natural law is in itself of the greatest assistance in accomplishing results.

COMPARATIVE STATEMENT OF POST MORTEM FINDINGS IN DEATH BY STARVATION (MEDICAL), AND POST MORTEM FINDINGS IN DEATH DURING THE FAST AS NOTED IN THE TEXT.

EMACIATION:
DEATH BY STARVATION (MEDICAL): Marked.
DEATH DURING THE FAST: In cases where cirrhosed state of liver or stomach existed, emaciation was similar to that in chronic ailments, but in the other instances it was not at all marked.

SKIN:
DEATH BY STARVATION (MEDICAL): Shriveled and wrinkled; emits a fetid odor; sometimes dark brown vanishy coating; tightly adherent to parts beneath; rough scurvy surface.
DEATH DURING THE FAST: Smooth and pliable in all cases; free from odor; no coating; not adherent. Except in cases of cirrhosis of liver or stomach, perfectly white. In the latter sinused condition as noted.

SUB-CUTANEOUS FAT:
DEATH BY STARVATION (MEDICAL): Absent.
DEATH DURING THE FAST: In all cases sub-cutaneous fat was present. This was especially so where disintegration of the liver is noted.

POST MORTEM RIGIDITY:
DEATH BY STARVATION (MEDICAL): Pronounced.
DEATH DURING THE FAST: Very slight.

PUTREFACTION:
DEATH BY STARVATION (MEDICAL): Sets in at once and progresses very rapidly.
DEATH DURING THE FAST: Very slow in progress. No preservatives were used on any body before holding the autopsy. In one instance post mortem was held one month after death, and putrefaction was hardly noticeable. Slowness of decay is attributable to the constant employment of both external and internal baths during treatment. Fasting is a process of elimination in immediate result, and the products that tend to swift decomposition are removed from the body as rapidly as formed.

HEART:
DEATH BY STARVATION (MEDICAL): Usually contracted, containing only a small amount of blood. Sometimes distinct atrophy.

DEATH DURING THE FAST: Normal in all cases.

LUNGS:
DEATH BY STARVATION (MEDICAL): Normal but smaller.
DEATH DURING THE FAST: Normal except as noted.

BLOOD:
DEATH BY STARVATION (MEDICAL): Lessened in amount, but thin and fluid from anemia.
DEATH DURING THE FAST: Abundance of blood. No apparent anemia.

BLADDER:
DEATH BY STARVATION (MEDICAL): Invariable empty. Sometimes much atrophied.
DEATH DURING THE FAST: In all cases contained some water. Pus as noted. No atrophy except in CASE 7.

SPLEEN:
DEATH BY STARVATION (MEDICAL): Not noteworthy.
DEATH DURING THE FAST: Normal in majority of cases. Disintegration noted in CASE 4, atrophy in CASES 6 and 7.

PANCREAS:
DEATH BY STARVATION (MEDICAL): Always atrophied, sometimes to practical disappearance.
DEATH DURING THE FAST: Atrophy noted in CASES 6 and 7; hypertrophy with cirrhosis in CASE 4; incipient cirrhosis in CASES 10 and 11. Others normal.

OMENTUM:
DEATH BY STARVATION (MEDICAL): Transparent and destitute of fat.
DEATH DURING THE FAST: In all cases some fat; in CASE 4 excessive fat. Transparent in no case.

LIVER:
DEATH BY STARVATION (MEDICAL): Unaltered except in size, which is lessened.
DEATH DURING THE FAST: Noted in all cases. There were no general characteristics; the organ varied in size and structure with the individual.

GALL BLADDER:
DEATH BY STARVATION (MEDICAL): Usually full; contents staining adjacent tissues.
DEATH DURING THE FAST: CASE 8 was the only instance in which there was staining of adjacent tissues. Others were as noted or normal.

STOMACH:
DEATH BY STARVATION (MEDICAL): Small, contracted; walls thin; mucosa corrugated and pale.

DEATH DURING THE FAST: Several cases showed extreme dilation; two were in state of cirrhosis; none showed contractions except CASE 3 (hour-glass), and CASES 10 and 11 (cirrhosis). Other variations as noted.

INTESTINES:
DEATH BY STARVATION (MEDICAL): Show uniform contraction as to lumen and length; walls usually thin and transparent to light; their atrophy in this connection is characteristic. Sometimes empty; sometimes containing dark mucus; sometimes distended with gas.
DEATH DURING THE FAST: The condition of the intestines is specifically noted in all cases. There were no general characteristics, but in no instance were the walls unduly thin.0

KIDNEYS:
DEATH BY STARVATION (MEDICAL): Do not seem to suffer.
DEATH DURING THE FAST: Suffered as noted.

One fact of significance shown in the postmortem findings and in the comparison noted above is that, no matter how general were the defects in other organs, nor how emaciated the body, unless they themselves were organically imperfect, the heart, the lungs, and the brain were normal in size and in functional ability. It may be added that, although not always specifically stated, the brain in each instance in the cases cited was thoroughly dissected.

Through the facts related, the immediate cause of death in every instance quoted can easily be traced to its origin. Organic deficiency is the direct result of functional digestive impairment. The scientific worth of this observation is much enhanced by the fact that in these autopsies the organs were presented unaffected by recent drug paralysis. The cases that exhibited glands that were hardened or atrophied were invariably of an emaciated or wiry physique, while those in which a softening of the organs had occurred were inclined to obesity. It is also interesting to note that, where mental control was lacking at any stage of the fast, the colon at dissection showed displacement and distortion that rendered evacuation of its contents almost impossible, even with enemata.

From the scientific viewpoint the observations included in the present chapter are undoubtedly of greatest import in the text. By them the theory of Fasting for the Cure of Disease is substantiated as a fact, and proof of its efficacy as a remedy is rendered incontrovertible.

CHAPTER XIX: SCHOOLS OF NATURAL HEALING

'Science does its duty, not in telling us the causes of spots in the sun, but in explaining to us the laws of our own life, and the consequences of their violation.'

Ruskin

As elsewhere expressed, the fast in itself is but a means to an end, but by its use in the treatment of disease, many mechanical defects in organs are entirely overcome through muscular rest and relaxation. Certain accessories are, however, brought into play. Bodily cleanliness and sanitation are essential, and mechanical adjustment of bones, muscular manipulation, and the internal bath are all invaluable concomitants of treatment.

In connection with muscular manipulation and bone adjustment, two distinct schools of healing have arisen in late years, those of Osteopathy and Chiropractic.

Osteopathy is defined as "that science or system of healing which treats disease of the human body by manual therapeutics for the stimulation of the remedial forces within the body itself, for the correction of misplaced tissue, and for the removal of obstructions or interferences with the fluids of the body, all without the internal administration of drugs or medicine." The name, derived as it is from the Greek, osteon, bone, and pathos, suffering, is not such a misnomer as might at first appear. The osteopathic theory is that many disease symptoms originate in bony lesions. This applies more particularly to the vertebral column, which, owing to its complex mechanism, is liable to several forms of sub-dislocation, depending upon the region in which they may occur. The most common is that of rotation followed by forward or backward displacement of a single vertebra. Compensation always succeeds these changes so that the disturbance is communicated to the ones above or below, thus forming a group. These lesions are detected by the touch and are verified by tenderness of the surrounding parts. They are necessarily slight, but the theory supposes them sufficient to profoundly influence adjacent tissue.

Mobility of the spine is of first importance, for in health there is motion between adjacent vertebrae. Lack of movement may be caused by muscular tension, by stretching of ligaments, or by a union of the parts due to bony deposit. Following any of these conditions, the theory holds, are functional or organic disturbances, acute becoming chronic. Nerves are pinched or impinged, and, as the circulation of the blood to an organ depends upon its nerve control, organic mechanism is interfered with, and disease begins.

Chiropractics is defined as "a system of therapeutic treatment for disease through the adjustment of the articulations of the human body, particularly those of the spine, with the object of relieving pressure or tension upon nerve filaments." As in Osteopathy, the operations are performed with the hands, no drugs being administered.

The two theories above presented are seen to be most closely related. But, it must be obvious that each school is reasoning from effect to cause when the claim is advanced that spinal lesions primarily lower nutrition. Muscles built when a state of mal-nutrition exists are not adequate for the work of supporting the bony structure with the delicate adjustment that combines strength with the necessary degree of flexibility. Barring displacement of vertebrae through an accident that forcibly disturbs the arrangement of the separate bones of the spinal column, there is but one source from which may arise a condition of lowered nutrition in any one of the muscles of the body impaired digestion. Perfect digestion insures perfect nutrition, and perfect nutrition must conserve muscular tone.

Both Osteopathy and Chiropractics are cut short of their greatest possibilities when they are applied apart from the fast. In the presence of a full stomach they become mere methods of force and stimulation, which, in many respects, are detrimental to health. They are then to be classed only as passive physical culture, in which the patient permits the operators to exercise the muscles instead of working them himself. During a fast, all muscles of the body are in a state of perfect relaxation, a natural result of the process of rest and elimination in progress. They respond in this condition to every impetus, and blood circulation at the same time is directly amenable to the stimulation applied. Hence the value, both local and general, of a combination with the fast of Osteopathic manipulation and Chiropractic thrust.

In pregnancy and confinement osteopathic methods are superior to all others in equalizing circulation and in facilitating delivery. In correcting uterine displacement, fasting removes congestion, relaxes the parts, and manual adjustment completes the cure. Manipulation at all times is an aid to elimination, but especially is this so during the fast; and, when a patient is weak and despondent, circulation, thus stimulated, buoys. Congested glands that so often suppurate and develop into false or true cancerous growths may, through manipulation, be caused to dis- appear by the increased power of absorption thus induced. This applies to all local swellings and excrescences, the operation compelling natural augmentation of blood in the parts.

Osteopathy and Chiropractics are purely mechanical accessories in the treatment of disease, and, as such, their field of practice is limited. But, in connection with the method outlined in the text, their efficiency is largely extended, and, used in conjunction, the three schools form a perfect combination for the prevention and cure of disease.

Christian Science ranges itself with the various theories of psycho-therapy that have been advanced from time to time, but its effect in the treatment of disease is of worth only as regards the suggestive power of mind over matter. It, with other similar cults, neglects the physical body and its functions, and calls upon the soul to further its ends. The interdependence of matter and mind is the subject of detailed discussion in another chapter, and need not be repeated here. Healing the sick as well as the sinful is an ideal union in purpose. Needless to say, it is seldom found in practice, yet there is truth in the thought that physical health is a prime factor in the process of attaining spiritual excellence.

All practical working schools that employ natural aids to health in their operation are mutually concerned in the conservation of physical balance in man. Excluding the quasi-science of medicine, with the exception of its rarely needed surgical branch, the methods of natural healing enumerated embody a perfect combination.

(THE END)

GLOSSARY

ABDOMEN: The belly.
ABERRATION: A wandering from.
ABEYANT: Absence; suspension.
ABSCESS: A cavity containing pus.
ABSORPTION: The sucking in or taking up of a fluid by anything.
ABSTINENCE: Voluntary privation or self-denial in diet, etc.
ACCOUCHEMENT: Confinement, lying-in, delivery.
ACCRUE: To arise, to be added to.
ACETONE: A chemical compound developed in the body by fermentation of organic matters.
ACID: As adjective, sour, tart. As noun, a compound of the gas, hydrogen, with other substances.
ADDENDUM: A thing to be added.
ADENOID: A growth that resembles a gland.
ADHERENT: Sticking to or grown to a surface.
ADIPOSE: Fatty.
ADJACENT: Lying near to.
ADOLESCENCE: The period between puberty and maturity.
ALIENIST: One who treats mental disease.
ALIMENTARY CANAL: The digestive tube and accessory glands.
ALKALINE: A salt of any kind that effervesces with acids; the opposite of an acid.
ALLEVIATE: To lessen, to diminish, to allay.
AMELIORATE: To make better.
ANEMIA: A deficiency of blood and red corpuscles.
ANEMIC: Pertaining to anemia.
ANAESTHETIC: A substance producing insensibility or unconsciousness.
ANALOGY: Similarity of relations between one thing and another.
ANTISEPTIC: Preventing or destroying putrefaction.
ANUS: The lower opening of the alimentary canal.
APATHY: Deadness of the emotions, want of feeling.
APERIENT: A gentle purgative.
APOPLEXY: Paralysis from rupture of a blood vessel in the brain.
APPENDICITIS: Inflammation of the vermiform appendix.
APPENDIX (VERMIFORM): The worm-shaped appendage to the cecum.
ARTICULATION: A joint.
ASPHYXIATION: The condition caused by non-oxygenation of the blood; suffocation.
ASSIMILATION: The act of absorbing nutriment, and its change into tissue, blood, etc.
ATROPHY: The wasting of a part from lack of nutrition.
AUGMENTATION: The act of increasing.
AUTO-INTOXICATION: Self-poisoning.

AUTOPSY: The examination of a body after death.
AUTO-TOXIN: Any poisonous substance originating within the body.
AXIOM: A self-evident truth.
BACILLI: The plural of bacillus.
BACILLUS: Any one of a genus of rod-like organisms, microscopic in size.
BACTERIA: The microscopic organisms that cause putrefaction; microbes; bodies similar to bacilli, but differing in form.
BANEFUL: Harmful, poisonous.
BARRENNESS: The state of being incapable of producing offspring.
BILE: The yellow, bitter liquid secreted by the liver.
BIO-CHEMISTRY: The chemistry of living tissues.
BOLUS: Medicine made into the form of a pill.
BOUGIE: A slender cylindrical instrument, solid or hollow.
BOWEL: The intestine.
BLADDER: The membranous receptacle of the urine.
BRONCHIAL: Pertaining to the Bronchi or main branches of the Trachea.
BUOY: To support a person or his hopes.
BUTTOCKS: The rump, the protuberant part behind.
CALIBRE: The internal diameter of a rod or tube.
CANAL ALIMENTARY: The digestive tube and accessory glands.
CANCER: A malignant growth having a tendency to spread.
CANKER: An eating sore, especially in the mouth.
CAPILLARY: A minute blood vessel.
CAPSULE: A soluble shell for administering medicine.
CARBOHYDRATE: A compound of carbon with hydrogen and oxygen, the latter gases being in proportion to form water.
CARBONIC ACID: A pungent, suffocating gas, the product of respiration.
CARDIAC OPENING: The upper opening of the stomach, so-called because nearest the heart.
CARTILAGINOUS: Of the nature of cartilage or gristle.
CATARRHAL: Of the nature of catarrh, which is an inflammation of the mucus membrane.
CATEGORY: A list or class.
CATHARTIC: A purgative medicine.
CAUTERIZE: To burn or sear with substances or instruments.
CECUM: The blind pouch at the head of the large intestine.
CELIBATE: One who is unmarried.
CHOLAGOGUE: A medicine that promotes the flow of bile.
CHYLE: The milky fluid of intestinal digestion.
CIRCULATORY: Pertaining to the circulation of the blood.
CIRRHOSED: Pertaining to cirrhosis.
CIRRHOSIS: Thickening of the connective tissue of an organ.
CLINICAL: Pertaining to a sick-bed or clinic.
CLOT: A mass of thickened blood.

COAGULATED: Thickened (as of fluids), curded.
CODEIN: One of the alkaloids derived from opium.
COLIC: Spasmodic pain in the abdomen.
COLLATERAL: Accompanying, aiding.
COLON: The superior part of the large intestine.
COLON TUBE: A long rubber tube for insertion through anus and sigmoid flexure into the colon.
COMA: An abnormally deep sleep; stupor.
COMATOSE: In a condition of coma.
COMMENSURATE: Having the same measure or extent; equal, proportional.
COMMINUTION: The process of breaking into pieces.
CONCOMITANT: Accompanying; existing in conjunction with.
CONDIGN: Adequate, deserved.
CONGENITAL: Existing from birth; innate.
CONGESTION: Excess of blood in a part.
CONSERVE: To preserve or protect from injury or loss.
CONSTIPATION: Sluggish action of the bowels.
CONTAGION: The communication of disease by contact.
CONTINENT: Complete abstinence from indulgence in sexual intercourse.
CONVALESCENCE: The period of recovery after disease.
COORDINATION: Harmonious action, as of muscles.
CORD, SPINAL: The cord of nerve tissue in the canal of the spinal column.
CORD, UMBILICAL: The navel-string attaching the fetus to the placenta or after-birth.
CORIUM: The deep layer of the skin.
CORROSIVE: A substance that eats away or destroys.
CORRUGATION: A contraction into wrinkles or folds.
CRISES: The plural of Crisis, a turning-point in any matter.
CRITERIA: The plural of Criterion, a standard by which anything is judged.
CROUPOUS: Pertaining to Croup, which is acute inflammation of the larynx and trachea.
CRUX: The cross, the central point.
CULT: A system of religious belief.
CURD: The coagulated or curdled part of milk, which is usually made into cheese.
CUTANEOUS: Pertaining to the skin.
CUTICLE: The epidermis or outer layer of the skin.
CYST: A membranous sack containing fluid.
DEBILITY: Weakness, loss or want of strength.
DECOMPOSITION: Putrefaction, decay.
DEGENERATE: Fallen off from a better to a worse state; declined in natural or moral worth.
DELIRIUM: Mental aberration due to disease.

DELIVERY: Parturition, child-birth.
DENSITY: The quality of being close or compact.
DENUDE: To make bare or naked.
DEPLETE: To reduce, to lessen.
DESIDERATA: Plural of Desideratum, a state of things to be desired.
DETERIORATION: The act of reducing anything in value or quality.
DETRIMENTAL: Causing hurt; injurious.
DIAGNOSIS: The recognition of disease from its symptoms.
DIAGNOSTICIAN: One skilled in diagnosing.
DIAPHRAGM: The muscular wall between the chest and the abdomen.
DIARRHEA: Excessive discharge of fluid evacuations from the bowels.
DIET: Food; a system of feeding.
DIETARY: Pertaining to diet; a system of feeding.
DIETETICS: The branch of treatment referring to diet.
DIETITIAN: One skilled in dietetics.
DIGESTION: Conversion of food into form suitable for assimilation.
DIGITALIS: Drug made from the poisonous plant, Foxglove, used as a heart stimulant.
DILATE: To enlarge in all directions.
DISINTEGRATION: The breaking-up of a body into its parts.
DISLOCATION: A displacement of organs or of the surfaces of the articulations or joints.
DISPARITY: Inequality.
DISSECT: To separate the parts of.
DISSOLUTION: Death.
DOGMA: A doctrine put forward to be received on the authority of the propounder.
DORSAL: Pertaining to the back; as to vertebrae, those lying between the neck and the loins.
DOUCHE: A stream of water directed upon a part.
DRASTIC: Powerful, acting with strength.
DUCT: A tube to convey a liquid.
DUODENUM: The first part of the small intestine.
DYSPEPSIA: Impaired or imperfect digestion.
EFFLUVIUM: An exhalation or vapor perceivable by the sense of smell.
e.g.: For example.
EJECT: To cast out.
ELIMINATION: The act of expelling, excreting, casting out.
EMACIATED: Thin from loss of flesh.
EMANATION: An effluvium; that which proceeds from a body.
EMBOLISM: The obstruction of a blood-vessel by a blood-clot.
EMETIC: A substance that causes vomiting.
EMPIRICAL: Depending upon experience or observation.
ENEMA: A liquid injected into the rectum.

ENEMATA: The plural of Enema.
EPICURE: One who gives himself up to the enjoyments of the table.
EPIDEMIC: Common to many people; a prevailing ailment.
EPILEPSY: Falling sickness; a nervous affection with loss of consciousness and convulsions.
EQUILIBRIUM: A state of balance.
ERADICATE: To root out; to exterminate.
EROTIC: Pertaining to sexual passion.
ETHER: The subtle fluid filling all space; also a colorless fluid used as an anesthetic.
EVACUATION: The act of causing a discharge from any of the excretory passages.
EVAPORATION: The process of turning into vapor.
EXCRESCENCE: An abnormal outgrowth of the body.
EXCRETE: To throw off worn-out material.
EXPECTORATION: The process of ejecting matter from the lungs or trachea by spitting.
EXTIRPATE: To cut out or off; to eradicate.
EXTRA-UTERINE: Outside the uterus.
EXUDATION: The state of being emitted like moisture through the pores.
FALLACY: That which deceives or misleads the eye or the mind.
FALLOPIAN TUBE: One of the two small tubes on each side of the uterus that convey the ova from the ovaries.
FANATICISM: Extravagant notions or opinions.
FECAL: Pertaining to the discharge of the bowels.
FECES: The discharge of the bowels.
FERMENT: To change by chemical action.
FETID: Having an offensive smell.
FETUS: The young in the womb after it is perfectly formed, i. e., after the fourth month of gestation.
FICTITIOUS: Imaginary, false, not real.
FILAMENT: A thread-like structure.
FILTER: To strain from solid particles.
FLEXIBILITY: The quality of being easily bent.
FLUCTUATING: A rising and falling suddenly; unsteadiness.
FOCUS: The meeting-point of reflected or refracted rays of light.
FOMENTATION: The application of warm liquids to the body.
FUNCTION: The normal or special action of a part.
GALL-BLADDER | GALL-CYST | GALL-SAC: The pear-shaped sac in the right lobe of the liver, the reservoir for the bile.
GALL-STONES: Stones built up of layers of carbonate of lime in the gall-bladder and its ducts.
GANGLIA: Plural of Ganglion, a sub-nerve center.
GANGRENE: The mortification or death of soft tissue.

GASTRIC: Pertaining to the stomach.
GELATINOUS: Resembling gelatin; jelly-like.
GENITAL: Pertaining to the organs of generation.
GERM: A microbe or bacterium.
GERMICIDE: An agent destroying germs.
GESTATION: The act of carrying young in the uterus from the time of conception to that of delivery.
GLAND: A secretory organ.
GLEET: Chronic state of gonorrhea with discharge.
GONOCOCCUS: The specific germ of gonorrhea.
GONORRHEA: A contagious inflammation with discharge from the genital organs.
GRANULATION Formation of small elevations on a healing surface.
HEART: The hollow muscular body, the center of the circulatory system.
HEMISPHERE: Half a sphere; as to the brain, one of the upper spheroidal portions.
HEMORRHAGE: A flow of blood from the vessels.
HICCOUGH: A sudden inspiration followed by expiration accompanied by a noise.
HYGIENE: The science of health.
HYPERTROPHY: Abnormal increase in size of a part or an organ.
HYPOCHONDRIAC: One affected with morbid anxiety regarding the health.
HYPOTHESIS: A supposition.
HYSTERIA: A nervous disorder of females with innumerable symptoms of an emotional nature.
ILEO-CECAL: Pertaining to the Ileum and Cecum.
ILEUM: The lower half of the small intestine.
IMBIBED: Taken in by drinking.
IMMUNITY: Freedom from risk of infection.
IMPACTED: Wedged in.
IMPEDE: To hinder; to obstruct.
IMPETUS: The force with which any body is driven or impelled.
IMPINGE: Literally, to fall against; in Osteopathy used with reference to nerves pinched between adjacent vertebrae.
IMPOTENCE: A lack of sexual power.
INANITION: Exhaustion arising from organic inability to assimilate food.
INCEPTION: The beginning.
INCOHERENCY: The quality of being unconnected in ideas, speech, etc.
INCREMENT: Increase or growth.
INCUMBENT: Resting upon one as a duty or obligation.
INDICES: Plural of Index, that which serves to point out.
INDUBITABLE: Not to be doubted.
INFECTION: The communication of disease-germs.
INFILTERING: Sifting in, or filtering in.

INFLUX: An inflow.
INGEST: To introduce food into the body by the mouth.
INHALE: To draw into the lungs.
INJECTION: Forcing of liquid into a cavity or vessel of the body.
INSALIVATE: To mix food with saliva during mastication.
INSIDIOUS: Sly, treacherous.
INTENTION: The process of healing.
INTERIM: The meantime; the intervening time or period.
INTERMITTENT: Occurring at intervals.
INTERSTICES: Spaces; intervals; pores.
INTUSSUSCEPTED: One part slipped into another, said of the intestines.
ITERATION: Repetition; the act of repeating.
JEJUNUM: The second portion of the small intestine of which it forms two-fifths.
JUGULAR: Pertaining to the neck. The jugular veins are three in number; their office is to return the blood from the head.
KATABOLISM: A retrograde change in the tissues of the body.
KIDNEYS: The organs secreting urine.
LARYNX: The upper part of the windpipe; the organ of voice.
LASCIVIOUS: Lewd, lustful.
LASSITUDE: Weakness, exhaustion.
LESION: Structural tissue change from injury or disease.
LEUCORRHEA: A whitish discharge from the vagina.
LIGAMENT: A band of fibrous tissue binding parts together.
LIVER: The largest glandular organ of the body, secreting bile.
LOBE: A rounded division of an organ.
LOCOMOTOR ATAXIA: A peculiar form of apparent paralysis with unsteady and disorderly muscular movements.
LONGEVITY: Long life.
LUBRICANT: A substance producing slipperiness, usually an oil or a grease.
LUMEN: The caliber of a tube, as of the bowels or blood-vessels.
LUNGS: The organs of respiration.
MALIGNANT: Virulent; fatal.
MALNUTRITION: Poor nutrition.
MAMMALS: Animals who suckle their young.
MANDATORY: Containing an order or command.
MANIA: Delirium or madness.
MANIPULATION: Treatment with the hands; handling.
MASSAGE: Manipulation; methodic pressure, friction, and kneading of the body.
MASTICATION: The process of chewing.
MASTURBATION: The production of the sexual orgasm in a manner other than natural.
MAXIMUM: The greatest quantity.

MEDIUM: That in which anything lives; surrounding conditions.
MELANCHOLIA: Depression of spirits; gloominess.
MEMBRANE: A thin enveloping or lining substance.
MENOPAUSE: The end of the menstrual life; the change of life.
MENSES: The monthly flow from the womb.
MENSTRUAL: Pertaining to the menses.
MESENTERY: The membrane which forms the attachment between the small intestines and the abdomen.
METABOLISM: A change in the intimate condition of cells, constructive or destructive.
MICROBE: Any minute or micro-organism.
MICRO-ORGANISM: A minute organism.
MINIMUM: The smallest quantity.
MISNOMER: A mistaken or misapplied name.
MITIGATION: The process of making milder or abating.
MITRAL: Miter-like; applied to the valve situated at the left auricular opening of the heart.
MOBILITY: The property of being easily moved.
MORBID: Not healthy; diseased; pertaining to disease.
MORTALITY: The death rate; the state of being mortal.
MOTOR: Applied to muscles and nerves moving a part.
MUCOSA: A mucus membrane.
MUCUS: The viscid liquid secretion of mucus membrane.
MUTATION: The act of changing; change.
MYOPIA: Near-sightedness.
MYOPIC: Pertaining to Myopia.
NARCOTIC: Medicine that produces sleep or torpor.
NASAL: Pertaining to the nose.
NAUSEA: Sickness at the stomach; a desire to vomit.
NAVEL: The narrow and deep impression in the center of the abdomen, marking where the fetus was attached to the placenta by the umbilical cord; the umbilicus.
NEUTRALIZE: To render negative or inactive.
NOSTRILS: The two apertures or cavities in the nose which give passage to the air and to the secretions of the nose.
NOSTRUM: A secret formula for a medicine, and the medicine itself.
NOXIOUS: Harmful; poisonous.
NUTRIENT: A nutritious substance; conveying nutriment.
NUTRITION: The process of assimilation of food.
NUTRITIVE: Affording nutrition.
OBESITY: Fatness; corpulence.
OCCLUDE: To block up.
OMENTUM: A fold of the peritoneum connecting the abdominal viscera with the stomach.

OPIATE: A medicine compounded with opium; a narcotic.
ORIFICE: A mouth or entrance; an opening.
ORTHODOX: In accordance with that commonly held as true.
OS: A mouth; as to the uterus, its opening into the vagina.
OVARY: The organ of generation in the female, producing the ova or eggs.
OVUM: The female reproductive cell; an egg. Plural, Ova.
OXYGEN: One of the gaseous elements; the supporter of life and combustion.
PABULUM: Food; anything nutritive.
PACK: A moist towel or blanket placed on a patient.
PALPATION: Exploration with the hand.
PANCREAS: A digestive gland in the abdomen; the sweetbread.
PARADOXICAL: Inclined to notions seemingly impossible.
PARALYSIS: Loss of sensation or voluntary motion.
PARASITE: An organism that inhabits another organism and obtains nourishment from it.
PASTEURIZE: To destroy the microbic life by heating the substance.
PELVIS: The bony basin at the lower part of the trunk.
PER: A Latin preposition having the force of, passage through, by.
PERIOSTEUM: A dense lining membrane covering the surface of the bones of the body.
PERISTALSIS: The worm-like motion of the bowels, causing downward movement of their contents.
PERITONEUM: The membrane lining the inner surface of the abdomen.
PERITONITIS: Inflammation of the Peritoneum.
PERMEATE: To pass through the pores of.
PERNICIOUS: Highly destructive; fatal.
PHARYNX: The muscular membranous sac behind the mouth.
PHYSIOLOGY: The science of the functions of the body.
PHYSIQUE: The physical structure of an individual.
PICKET-LINE: A line of guards posted in front of an army to give notice of the approach of the enemy.
PLEURAL: Pertaining to the Pleura or membrane enveloping the lungs.
PLIABLE: Easily bent.
PNEUMOGASTRIC: Pertaining to the lungs and the stomach.
POLEMICAL: Argumentative; controversial.
PNEUMONIA: Inflammation of the lungs.
PORE: A small opening in the skin.
PORTAL: Pertaining to the Portal Vein which carries the blood to the liver.
POST MORTEM: Occurring after death.
POST NATAL: Occurring after birth.
POTENTIAL: As adjective, powerful; as noun, possessing power.
PRECLUDE: To shut out; to stop.
PREGNANCY: The condition of being with child.

PRESCRIBE: To lay down rules or directions; to direct to be used as a remedy.
PRIMORDIAL: First in order; primary, original.
PRISTINE: Belonging to an early period or state; original, primitive.
PROCREATION: Reproduction, generation.
PROGNOSIS: Prediction of course and end of disease.
PROLAPSED: Fallen down.
PROPAGATE: To generate; to produce.
PROSTATE: A glandular body situated around the neck of the bladder in the male.
PROTEID: An albuminoid constituent of an organism.
PROTEIN: The sulfur-free residue of a proteid after the action of caustic potash.
PROTOPLASM: Primitive organic cell-matter; germinal matter.
PSORIASIS: A chronic inflammatory skin-disease with scale formation.
PSYCHO-THERAPY: The treatment of disease by mental influence.
PUBERTY: The age of capability of reproduction.
PULSATION: A beating or throbbing sensation.
PULSE: The beat or shock felt in any artery when slight pressure is made on it, caused by the contraction of the heart.
PURGATIVE: A substance causing watery evacuations from the bowels; a cathartic.
PUS: A thick yellow fluid, the product of suppuration.
PUTREFY: To cause to rot or decay with an offensive odor.
PYLORUS: The opening of the stomach into the duodenum.
PYORRHEA: A discharge of pus, usually associated with the sockets of the teeth.
QUASI: Almost; something which resembles.
QUOTA: A proportional share or part.
RASH: An eruption on the skin.
RATION: A stated or fixed amount; an allowance.
RATIONAL: Reasonable.
RATIONALE: A statement of reasons.
RECIPROCAL: Mutual; mutually interchangeable.
RECTUM: The lower part of the large intestine.
RECUMBENT: Reclining; lying.
RECUPERATION: Return to health; convalescence.
RECUR: To occur again; to be repeated after intervals.
REFLEX: An involuntary action from nerve-stimulus.
REFUTE: To prove to be false or erroneous.
REGIME: Mode or system of rule or management.
REGIMEN: The methodic use of food.
REGURGITATION: The flowing back into the vessels of the heart of the blood which has just left them.

RELAXATION: Absence of tension, usually with reference to the muscles.
REMEDY: An agent used in the treatment of disease.
REPLICA: A copy of an original.
RESIDUE: That which remains.
RESPIRATION: Inspiration and exhalation of air by the lungs.
RHEUMATISM: A disease symptom with fever, pain, inflammation and swelling of the joints.
RIGIDITY: Stiffness; immobility.
ROTARY: Having a motion on its axis like a wheel.
ROTATION: Turning on the axis.
RUDIMENT: That which is unformed or undeveloped.
SACRUM: Five vertebrae at the lower extremity of the spinal column that rapidly diminish in size from above downwards and are united into one mass in the adult.
SALISBURY TREATMENT: A system of treatment employing meat and hot water.
SALIVARY: Pertaining to the saliva.
SALIVATION: An excessive secretion of saliva.
SALPINGITIS: Inflammation of a Fallopian tube.
SALUTARY: Promotive of health.
SATURATION: The condition of holding in solution all of a solid capable of being contained.
SCROFULA: A constitutional condition with glandular tumors and a tuberculous tendency.
SCURVY: Affected or covered with scurf or scabs.
SECRETE: To separate from the blood.
SENSORY: Pertaining to sensation.
SENSUAL: Pertaining to the senses or bodily organs of perception.
SEPTIC: Relating to putrefaction.
SEPTICEMIA: A morbid condition from the absorption of septic products.
SEQUENCE: A following or coming after; succession.
SEROUS: Having the nature of serum.
SERUM: The fluid constituent of the blood.
SIGMOID FLEXURE: The S-shaped portion of the colon above the rectum.
SIMULATE: To assume the likeness of; to feign, to counterfeit.
SINUS: A hollow. In Anatomy the term is applied especially to a dilated vein or receptacle of blood.
SITZ-BATH: A bath in a sitting posture.
SLOUGH: To separate from the living part, as the dead part in mortification.
SOPHISTICATED: Not genuine.
SPECTRA: Colors.
SPINAL CORD: The cord of nerve tissue in the canal of the spinal column.
SPINE: The vertebral column.

SPLEEN: An oval organ behind the outer end of the stomach. Its use is unknown.
SPLINT: A support to hold fractured bones or inflamed joints rigid.
SPUTUM: Expectorated matter.
STERILIZED: Subjected to heat of sufficient intensity to destroy germ life.
STERTOROUS: Breathing with a sonorous sound.
STIMULATION: The act of exciting; a quickly diffused but transient increase of vital energy.
STIMULUS: Anything exciting an organ.
STOMACH: The chief digestive organ of the body.
STRICTURE: A contraction of a duct or tube. The text refers to stricture of the urethra.
STRYCHNINE: A highly poisonous alkaloid made from Nux Vomica.
STULTIFACTION: Rendering worthless.
STUPEFY: To make dull or dead to external influences.
SUBCUTANEOUS: Under the skin.
SUBJACENT: Underlying.
SUBSERVIENT: Acting as a subordinate instrument.
SUBVERSIVE: Tending to overthrow.
SUDORIFEROUS: Carrying sweat.
SUPERFICIAL: Confined to the surface.
SUPERSEDE: To displace.
SUPERVENING: To take place; to happen; to occur.
SUPPURATING: Forming pus.
SUSTENANCE: That which supports life; food.
SYMPTOM: A sign of disease.
SYPHILIS: A chronic, infectious, venereal disease, which may also be hereditary, inducing cutaneous and other lesions.
TARTAR: The deposit of calcareous matter upon the teeth.
TENSION: The state of being stretched.
TENTATIVE: Based on experiment.
TERM: A definite period, as the full Term of gestation.
THERAPEUTICS: Science concerned with the application of remedies and the treatment of disease.
TISSUE: An aggregation of similar cells and fibers, forming a distinct structure.
TITILLATION: The act or sensation of tickling.
TONIC: An agent to produce normal tone of an organ or a part.
TONSIL: A glandular organ on each side of the throat.
TONSILITIS: Inflammation of the tonsils.
TOXICATION: The process of cumulative poisoning from septic products.
TOXIN: A poison formed by bacteria in both living tissues and dead substances.
TRACHEA: The windpipe.

TREMOR: Involuntary trembling.
TRUNK: The body except the head and the limbs.
TUBERCLE: A small nodule of glandular cells constituting the condition called tuberculosis.
TUBERCULAR: Pertaining to or containing tubercles.
TUBERCULOSIS: An infectious disease due to a specific bacillus, characterized by the formation of tubercles.
TYPHOID: Resembling typhus. Typhoid fever is a continued acute, infectious fever, with intestinal lesions, etc.
ULCER: Suppuration upon a free surface; an open sore.
UMBILICAL CORD: The navel-string attaching the fetus to the placenta or after-birth.
UMBILICUS: The narrow and deep impression in the center of the abdomen, marking where the fetus was attached to the placenta by the navel-string; the navel.
UNITY: The state or condition of being one; oneness; singleness.
URETER: A tube carrying urine from kidney to bladder.
URETHRA: The excretory canal of the bladder.
URETHRITIS: Inflammation of the urethra.
URIC: Contained in or derived from urea, which is the chief solid constituent of urine, and is the principal waste product of tissue-decomposition.
URINE: The excretion of the kidneys.
UTERUS: The hollow muscular organ of the female generative system in which the fetus is contained during pregnancy.
VAGINA: The canal from the vulva to the uterus.
VALVULAR: Pertaining to a valve.
VEGETARIAN: One whose diet is vegetable.
VENEREAL: Pertaining to sexual intercourse.
VENOUS: Pertaining to a vein as opposed to an artery.
VERITY: The quality or state of being true; truth.
VERTEBRA: A bony segment of the spinal column. Plural, Vertebrae.
VICE VERSA: The reverse; the terms of the case being reversed.
VIRULENCE: The quality or state of being extremely poisonous.
VIRUS: Any organic poison; the pus from an ulcer; the result of some morbid action on the system.
VISCERA: The contents of the body cavities.
VISCID: Glutinous; ropy.
VISCOUS: The same as Viscid.
VISUAL: Pertaining to vision.
VITIATE: To taint; to infect.
VITUPERATION: Abuse. Viz. To, wit; namely; that is.
VOLITION: The will to act.
VULVA: The external female genitals.

WET-NURSE: A woman who suckles the child of another.
WHEY: The liquid part of milk separating from the curd in coagulation.
WOMB: The Uterus.

CPSIA information can be obtained
at www.ICGtesting.com
Printed in the USA
FSOW04n2042030216
16556FS